FOOD FIGHT

FOOD FIGHT

HOW WHAT WE EAT IS WEAPONIZED

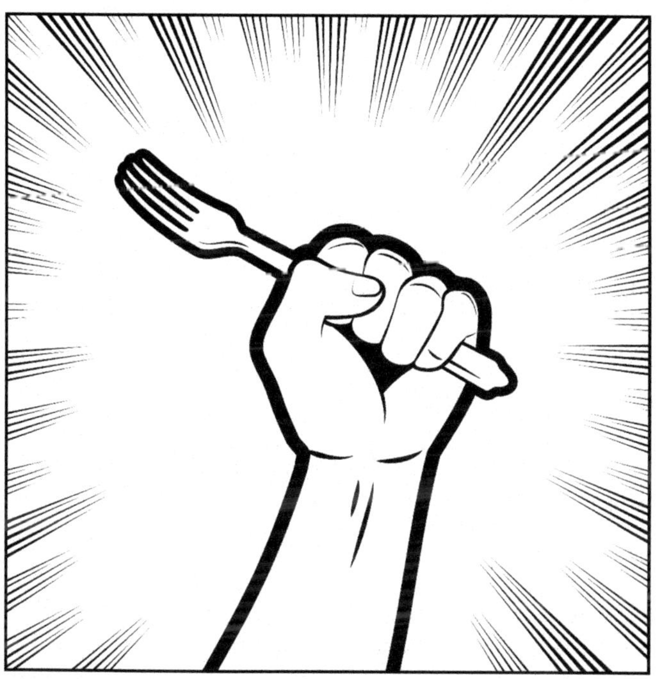

Edited by Miguel A. De La Torre

The Pilgrim Press, 1300 East 9th Street
Cleveland, Ohio 44114
thepilgrimpress.com

Published 2025.

Printed on acid-free paper.

Library of Congress Cataloging-in-Publication Data on file.
LCCN: 2024949588

ISBN 978-0-8298-0072-2 (paper)
ISBN 978-0-8298-0073-9 (ebook)

Printed in The United States of America.

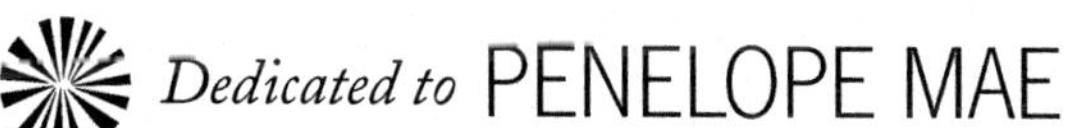
Dedicated to PENELOPE MAE

Contents

Section III—Africa

Section IV—South Asian Subcontinent

Section V—Southeast Asia

Section VI—Oceania

Preface

I DEDICATED THE PREVIOUS VOLUME of this series (*Shifting Climates, Shifting People*) to my firstborn grandchild. As I was finishing this book, my second grandchild, Penelope Mae, was born. She was born healthy just a few months after I had submitted the manuscript to the publishing house. They say we taste eternity through our grandchildren, as our DNA and memories of us continue to exist on planet earth way after we return to the dust from which we came. Penelope Mae is just a few months old now, but I would do anything to ensure her joy and happiness. I have no doubt that others—who are parents, grandparents, and even great-grandparents—having also looked into the eyes of their future in the form of an innocent babe who is flesh-of-their-flesh and blood-of-their-blood, would also do anything and everything to contribute toward their progeny's fulfilling life and future.

And yet, as we know based on multiple empirical studies, by the time Penelope Mae is my age, she will be living in a world negatively impacted by this generation's apathy. Our negligence in taking the ecological devastation surrounding us seriously seems to indicate that we really do not care about our families and those who will represent us in the future. We may verbally express love for those who will carry our memories into the next century, but we are actually—through our lack of action—expressing that we really do not give a damn about them. As I struggle to try to understand this disconnect, it becomes obvious that those who profit from a status quo that degrades the environment have convinced so many through the politicians they keep in their pockets like loose change that climate change is a hoax and deregulation is the best possible solution.

While the book is dedicated to Penelope Mae, I am cognizant that it might be decades before she might read the concerns I held for her future. Maybe those who read it today will, out of the love they profess for the next generation, change so as to begin the earth's healing. How I hope the concerns raised today in this book will seem to have been an exaggeration when Penelope Mae finally reads them. But alas, I am hopeless. Our lack in taking these concerns seriously today will only exacerbate the situation tomorrow.

Around the time I discovered I was again going to be an *abuelo*, I was organizing an international conference on the intersection of food, the environment, and oppression. Individuals from around the world participated in the conference, sharing about how the production of food is directly linked to environmental degradation and/or disenfranchisement. Papers were presented from Oceana, Asia, the Indian subcontinent, Africa, and North and South America. We approached this interconnectedness through different cultural contexts from the Global South to learn from each other about points of convergence and differences. We all need food to exist. We live in a world with enough resources to feed the current population. And yet, most of the world's inhabitants are either hungry or live with food insecurity. Why? Who profits from these global arrangements of scarcity? How is what we eat weaponized to maintain global structures of oppression?

This conversation was made possible because of the commitment to ecojustice of the Iliff School of Theology in Denver. They raised the necessary funds to host the conference. As one who confesses their technological ineptness, I realized that participants from around the world could not be brought into the same virtual room if not for Michael McMillan.

Also, Rachel Hackenberg, and her commitment to the cause of an environmentally sound future, deserves gratitude for agreeing to publish this third book of the series. I am grateful to Adam Bresnahan, production editor, for his herculean work of getting the manuscript ready for publication. Finally, I lift up Penelope Mae, to whom this book is dedicated. May she live in a world that does not demonstrate our sins of omission when it comes to ecojustice. Instead, may we—convicted of our complicity with ecological degradation—turn from our ways and strive to make this a more inhabitable, thus better, world for those who will come after us.

INTRODUCTION
Food Sense(s): Decentering Anthropocentrism

Miguel A. De La Torre

EATING ACTIVATES THE SENSE OF TASTE. When the chemical compounds of food intersect with the ten to fifty receptor cells located on each of the ten thousand buds on our tongue, our throat, and the roof of our mouths, information is relayed to the brain to distinguish among sweetness, bitterness, saltiness, sourness, and umami-ness. Along with taste, other senses interact with the process: the appearance of what we eat, how it smells, how it feels, and the sound it makes in our mouths. This thing we ingest does not appear to us *ex nihilo*, for it has its own story, a history that has evolved and intertwined alongside the history or story of humans. All too often this thing eaten, this thing that nourishes human bodies and provides them with the necessary sustenance to live, has been weaponized to bring disenfranchisement and death. Humans may devour food, but food also devours humans.

How can food ever taste pleasing once we are cognizant of the long historical connection with blood-soaked oppression? What is the taste of historically rotted, poisonous food whose noxious exploitative fumes choke our very nostrils to the point where we cannot breathe? What if food has its own sense(s), its own agency, complete with its own story, its own history in which humans are the object? What if humans are not the center of the social narrative but objectified by food and those who profit from food? All too often, food as material is reduced to an inert receptacle that is subject to outside forces that provide it with purpose and meaning. But what if food is more than simply a thing, something material? What if it also has agency? Can the sense of food produce a disinherited feeling or perception by means of a dispossessing stimulus?

Food, in this book, is explored as a materialist narrative that, contrary to the modernist project, weaves together the human and the thing (food) while reversing the positions of subject and object. Decentering anthropocentrism reveals that, rather than humans eating food, food is a threat that consumes its objectified human. Food as thing may be among the most fundamental requirements for survival within Maslow's classic hierarchy of needs, a hierarchy that places self-actualization at the pinnacle; but for those who fall short, this hunger for base needs causes, creates, and continues transculturally disenfranchising structures that objectify the many. The global market economy that generates massive profits out of the basic human need to eat has historically been and continues to be responsible for much of the misery and death experienced by the world's dispossessed.

Human hunger informs the relationship humans develop for and with food, but food also informs what humans desire, affecting the idea of what they consider tasty or repulsive. This coevolutionary relationship grants food its own importance and agency without depriving humans—specifically, those objectified through the denial of their humanity—concepts like justice. In fact, the story or history of food and its weaponization provides an analytical prism by which to better grasp and understand how injustices against humans and nonhumans, culture (understood as human activity) and nature (which encompasses food and humans), came to be legitimized and normalized.

Those of us who speak Spanish translate history as *historia*. But this word is somewhat ambiguous, for it can also connotes "tale, story." *La historia*, the *story* of food, is the *history* of transculturation, which comprises different hybrid food narratives. Writing in Spanish, Cuban ethnographer

Fernando Ortiz (1881–1961) coined the term transculturation (*transculturación*). Transculturation was to be a counterpoint to acculturation, which signifies the net loss process of acquiring another culture, of assimilating the so-called less developed culture into the so-called superior one. He sought to describe the historical process of identity formation by studying the history of material things (sugar and tobacco), fraught, as it was, with conquest and resistance.

Ortiz's racist idea of Black Cubans as savages stood at the center of his observation of the polarization of Cuban society. In his work *Contrapunteo cubano del tabaco y el azúcar*, he expresses the normative gaze of Eurocubans and the polarity between Black and white Cubans through the concept of "the Cuban counterpoint." For him, "Tobacco and sugar contradict each other in economics and in the social; even when rigid moralists have been preoccupied with them when considering the course of their history, viewing one with mistrust and the other with favor" (1940a: 1–2). According to Ortiz, sugar was introduced to the Américas by Cristoforo Colombo during his second voyage; likewise, Colombo introduced tobacco to Europe.[1]

For Ortiz, half the island, like sugar, is sweet, refined, odorless and white, while the other half, like tobacco, is raw, pungent, bitter, aromatic, and dark. Tobacco requires constant care; sugar can look after itself. Tobacco poisons; sugar nourishes. Within the spiraling smoke of a good Cuban cigar exists something revolutionary. The tobacco's consuming anarchical flames protest oppression. Sugar, on the other hand, contains neither rebellion nor resentment. It is calm, quiet, beyond suspicion. Sugar is the work of the gods, a scientific gift of civilization. Tobacco is of the devil, a magic gift of the savage world (1940a: 5–15, 46). Ortiz writes:

> Tobacco is dark, from Black to *mulato*; sugar is clear, from *mulata* to white. Tobacco does not change color, born black and dies with the color of its race. Sugar changes its coloration, born brown and whitens itself; it is a syrupy *mulata* that being blackish abandons

1. In reality, sugar was introduced to Cuba in 1523 when La Casa de la Contratación of Seville provided the financial backing needed to transplant the sugar industry from its base in the Canary Islands.

> herself to popular taste and later she bleaches and refines herself so as to pass for white, traveling the whole world, reaching all mouths, and being paid better, climbs the dominating categories of the social ladder (1940a: 7).

Ortiz was the first to use the Cuban stew *ajiaco* as a transcultural metaphor to symbolize the formation of Cuban identity and how diverse ethnic and racial backgrounds—some deemed by him to be superior and some inferior—came into being. His usage of *ajiaco* did not indicate his belief that Cuban culture achieved complete integration; rather, the *ajiaco*, as a nonstable thing, is still simmering without reaching a full synthesis. He notes that the Taíno Indians provided *maíz*, *papa*, *malanga*, *boniato*, *yuca*, and *ají*. To this, Spaniards added *calabaza*, *carne de vaca*, and *nabo*, while the Chinese added Eastern spices. Africans contributed *ñame* and *plátanos*, and with their culinary foretaste, extracted a meaning from this froth beyond mere clever cooking. Examining this culinary transcultural mixture, Ortiz concludes that Cubans are "a *mestizaje* of kitchens, a *mestizaje* of races, a *mestizaje* of cultures, a dense broth of civilization that bubbles on the stove of the Caribbean" (1940b: 165–69).

Compare the *ajiaco* with the more common acculturation metaphor of the "melting pot," used within the United States to symbolize the coming together of different cultures and races. The North American melting pot represents an ideal of all immigrant groups arriving to the shores of the United States and being placed into a pot where they "melt down" into a new culture that nonetheless remains Anglo-Saxon in flavor and nature. Consider the 1914 ceremony established by Henry Ford—a notorious antisemite—for his Ford English School. The school, established for his diverse immigrant workforce, prepared them for US citizenship through civics and English language lessons. Upon graduation, the students would descend into a large melting pot wearing their native "costume," only to emerge on the other side dressed as an "American" waving the red, white, and blue. This melting pot, in which the scum rises to the top as those at the bottom get burnt, reinforces just one ingredient—white supremacy. Contrary to the acculturating melting pot, a transcultural *ajiaco* retains the unique flavors of its diverse roots while enriching the other elements.

Ingredients never fully dissolve, while others remain more distinct, easily recognizable within the hybridity stew. All provide flavor to the simmering *ajiaco*, a stew that by its very nature is always in a state of flux. For Ortiz, the people represented by these ingredients made a conscious decision to be rooted to a particular land. But did they?

Literary scholar Héctor Hoyos expands upon Ortiz's theoretical contribution with the concept of transcultural materialism, an intellectual praxis (as opposed to a philosophical doctrine) that is undergirded by a critique of extractivism—the exploitation of nature and labor. Rather than constituting two separate entities, nature and human labor, along with their histories, are intertwined. By studying nature as things, Hoyos demonstrates how social relationships intersect. He shows how things (in our case food) as objects are relegated to nonhuman entities and subservience to the preeminence of the human species. Transcultural materialism critiques the classic approach of natural history, which views humans as active and nature as passive. It is a praxis that considers "the noninstrumental use of stories and literary language to upset the nature-culture divide, affect our rapport with things, and reassess our place in human-nonhuman history" (2019, 3–4, 13, 199). For Hoyos, Ortiz defined his concept of transculturation during an age of eugenics and racism as the net loss of cultural exchange (acculturation) in the form of assimilation. Hoyos's usage of transcultural is thus positive and represents "a gain" (2019, 7).

Considering the personification of sugar and tobacco, I found Ortiz's usage of the term more ambiguous and problematic.[2] Through this transmutation of cultures, he argues that the combination of the diverse ingredients humans eat contributes to the formation of our identity. As a small child, I still recall that whenever my Cuban mother made an *ajiaco* from the scraps of leftovers, she would comment on its hearty qualities by stating: "*Hice un ajiaco que levanta los muertos.*"[3] For her and Ortiz, *ajiaco*, the mixture of our diverse roots, becomes a life-giving substance, something

2. This has not always been the case. Since the late 1990s, I also mistakenly maintained a positive interpretation of transculturation, specifically Ortiz's *ajiaco* metaphor, to signal a shared attempt to forge a new cooperative cultural reality.

3. I made an *ajiaco* that can raise the dead.

that can raise the dead (in life). But what if Ortiz and my beloved mother were wrong? What if the food that forms our identity is death-dealing? What if the diversity of foods consumes our diversity?

Ortiz's concept of transculturation is helpful for exploring this question because it denotes the imposition of the colonizer's culture on that of the colonized (Ortiz, 1940b, 98–99). With transculturation in Ortiz's sense, the full distinct aspects of marginalized cultures become erased under the weight of the ever-forming ethos "like sugar cane ground in the rollers of the mill" (1940b, 98). Like the assimilating term acculturation, transculturation also involves the crushing, the loss, the uprooting of the colonized culture and the dehumanization of its people (1940b, 102–103). Hence, transculturation, while better than acculturation, remains devastating to cultures as it masks power imbalances among the different *ajaico* ingredients.

Although I have reservations about transculturation, the hybrid in-between culture it creates, and the term's ambivalences that at once signify constructive and destructive practices, the term remains helpful for elucidating how a new reality (an *ajiaco*) can be created through the contact and mixing of diverse cultures, even if that contact can be violent. Hoyos's usage of the concept of transcultural materialism attempts to blur the lines between nature and culture. He "deploys storytelling [historytelling] as a form of political *and* ecological intervention" (2019, 88). Employing this insight, I suggest that by exploring food's *historia* we can discover why people are dehumanized by the weaponization of food. The critique of extractivism is key for analyzing the narrative of food as a material basis for culture, complete with its own agency. This, in turn, can contribute to the modern praxis toward liberation.

Studying the intersection of *las historias* (the stories or histories) of food as transculturation material and humans as material things can help explain how oppressive structures are developed and expanded. The autonomy attributed to the nonhuman should not be restricted to nature—or in the case of this book, food—but must be expanded to all living creatures who either depend on food as substance for existence, and to humans who must labor to bring food to market so a small elite can obtain profit, power, and privilege. Those who are marginalized as a consequence of the weaponization of food are relegated to and treated as nonhuman, subordinating their agency for a plate of lentils. By subjugating humans for needed food, the anthropocentrism of modernist history is challenged. The history of the relationship between food and humans involves the interrelation of nature and culture, illuminating how the exploitational forces and structures responsible for injustices faced by humans are the same exploitational forces and structure responsible for the use, abuse, and misuse of food.

This book explores the binding of human *historia* with the *historia* of food. Special attention is given to both the history/story of food as part of a nature whose economy situates it within culture and the history/story of humans oppressed by food and relegated to nonhuman things. An attempt is made to traverse nature and labor with the modernist concept of liberation through the power of retelling their story, their history. Liberation is here understood as restoring sense(s) to material things and restoring humanity to those made nonhuman by their labor. Liberation creates space within nature for ecological political action. The nonhuman agency of things like food is sought, becoming a conscious-raising method that privileges material things—nature that brings forth food and those whose humanity has been stolen. Against the modernist trend of separating culture and nature, this book therefore seeks to unite them in order to better comprehend the historical social forces that forged the identity of those relegated to the underside of history.

SECTION I

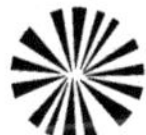

NORTH AMERICA

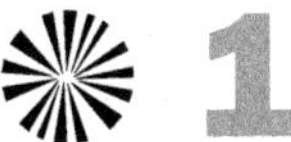 1

Three Sisters, Buffalo, Rice, and Salmon
Relationship or Max Profit?

Tink Tinker (wazhazhe udsethe/Osage Nation)

JUST SOUTH OF METRO denver[1] is Land that the local Native community calls its own piece of "Indian Country." Mandated by denver's city government in 1977, "Tall Bull memorial grounds" is a refuge for Native peoples of metro denver to enjoy community events and ceremonial activities. After 531 years of eurochristian invasion, colonization, and decimation of Turtle Island, Tall Bull is a protected place for Indians to fulfill their responsibilities with all of their Relations—the four-leggeds, winged, and all living and moving relatives. We take our fourteen-year-old daughter there to gather Medicine for ceremonies, demonstrating the reciprocal relationship we have with all our Relatives by offering Tobacco before picking a stalk of Sage. Buffalo is our daughter's close Relative to whom she pays attention throughout the year. The city of denver maintains a Buffalo herd by Tall Bull, and our daughter can visit with her Buffalo

1. All capitalization or lack thereof in this chapter is intentional.

cousins when she is out there. She is *toka tó*^{n}*wo*^{n}*gtho*^{n}, Buffalo clan, and has a Buffalo clan name. So important is that relationship and its responsibilities both to her clan and to the Osage People that Buffalo clan folk abstain from eating Buffalo meat, the protein that was central to the survival of the rest of an Osage village. Their job, as Buffalo clan, was always to protect that relationship of balance and harmony with the Buffalo Nation on behalf of the rest of the village. We eat Buffalo only because of the work done by the Buffalo clan to ensure our relationship is one of respect and Balance. This Balance is not an abstraction. It is a physical, tangible reality that is achieved and sustained by human action and cannot be mediated through the abstraction of words. My daughter abstains from eating Buffalo because they are her close Relatives, her siblings. So, when she moved into our home at the age of four, I made a promise that I would honor her and her clan by not eating Buffalo meat whenever she was with me or in our home.

Lest any eurochristian reader becomes glossy-eyed at a romanticized imagining of Native community assembling in their beads and feathers at Tall Bull for powwows and ceremonies, let me remind you that Tall Bull affords Native peoples only *seventy acres* to sustain relationships with all our Relatives. Before 1492, we could do that anywhere on Turtle Island. Indeed, eurochristian invasion and colonization has resulted in a state of war between human two-leggeds and all of our Relatives on this earth. Hence, we arrive in the twenty-first century with notions that food can be reduced to a weapon of war—no longer a Relative but now an object, a thing that can be used to distort and destroy the relationships that Native peoples have enjoyed with all living things since time immemorial.

As I think about the weaponization of food, I have to consider the deeper context of worldview difference and the forced imposition of the eurochristian worldview on Indigenous Peoples by the ongoing processes of colonialism. Like all Peoples around the world, American Indians have a historical and traditional relationship with certain foods. But the American Indian relationship with food goes far beyond issues of custom, recipes, taste, and the like. Indians have reciprocal and personal Relationships with the Plants and Animals that provide us with those traditional foods. Our Grandmothers—Corn, Beans, and Squash, the Three Sisters—were ubiquitous across Turtle Island, while Rice[2] was fundamentally important further north in the region called today the "great Lakes." Buffalo was a main source of protein across much of Turtle Island, and Salmon, for instance, provided that nutrient in the cuisine for Peoples of the northwest coast,[3] and whole communities move presciently out to the mouth of the river to greet Salmon ceremonially at the very moment they arrive to begin their ascent upstream for spawning.[4] These are just some of the foods that traditionally sustain Indigenous Peoples' lives on Turtle Island and with whom Natives maintain intentional interpersonal relationships.

In order to take the Land and commodify it into property, the colonizer had to work deliberately to break our relationships with those close Relatives that provide our food. The colonizer had to change our diets and our whole way of relating to food. They had to reduce us to wage labor dependent on the colonizer's own supply of objectified foodstuffs. They had to teach us to buy prepackaged groceries instead of making our reciprocal offerings before harvesting. Some of that history was inordinately violent, involving the burning of two-year stores of Corn in Iroquoian villages.[5] Today, even our eurochristian relatives can recognize the

---

2. Anishinaabeg people call it *manoomin*. The colonialists call it "wild rice" in english, but Native languages have no word for "wild." That word was used to disparage Native food sciences, just as it was used to disparage Indians and mark them as less-than eurochristian folk. Then, of course, it became a gourmet cuisine, and very expensive, option for colonialist tastes. But across the region where Rice grows naturally, it was a staple food item year-round. Harvesting was done by Natives in the fall with careful attention to making sure there would be future harvests.

3. Over the years of intense colonialist invasion, Native fishing for Salmon was increasingly criminalized—until court cases in the 1970s began to take Treaties (u.s constitution, article six: "highest law of the Land") more seriously. See the so-called boldt decision, 1974: united states v. washington, 384f. supp. 312 (w.d. wash. feb. 12, 1974).

4. See one description of this in kimmerer 2013, 234–237.

5. This wanton destruction happened in george washington's burned Earth tactic in his assault on Native Peoples opening up the western border to eurochristian Land-grabbing expansion (1776–1795). Using archival references, barbara alice mann reports these destructions in her book *george washington's war on Native America*, 2005.

violence committed against the Buffalo Nation.[6] In the 1870s, the u.s. army and well-to-do eurochristian tourists began exterminating millions of Buffalo, an act they determined was critical to the conquest of American Indians,[7] and some of the photos are really horrific.[8] The attack on Corn was different from the attack on Buffalos since it involved a longer, ongoing period of conversion to factory farming and hybridization of Corn. The changes always initiated desperation for Native folk. The relationships we learned to respect when we harvested food have become much more difficult as we buy cello-wrapped, pre-ground hamburger or canned and frozen vegetables in a modern supermarket, foods that have been mass-produced in the context of industrial farming. This process has damaged and continues to damage American Indian communities to this day, even when we might be able to afford purchasing this factory-food. As recently as 1994, the "north american free trade agreement" made the much cheaper north american hybrid corn crops available in mexico and central america to the extent that Indigenous farming became more economically untenable, threatening to reduce independent farmers to wage labor job markets in city centers.

A few years back, Q'eqchi' men in the rio polochic valley told me as they lost their own farming Land that they were forced to take jobs on huge plantations for the equivalent of about $1 per day to feed their families. During the thirty-six-year civil war (conflicto armado, 1963–1996) in guatemala, huge tracts of Land were converted to property and immediately cornered by the controlling rich families of the country, leaving less and less Land for guatemalan Indian Peoples to live on in any self-sufficiency. In this way, the country's elite, large property-owners, and international corporate factory farming have summarily converted Indigenous

---

6. See the new ken burns documentary: The american Buffalo, which began airing on pbs stations in october 2023.

7. See, for example, carol clark, "Buffalo slaughter left lasting impact on Indigenous Peoples," emory news center, emory university, august 23, 2023.

8. This link is to a famous photo of the time of a huge heap of buffalo skulls that were collected during this time of slaughter: https://en.wikipedia.org/wiki/File:Bison_skull_pile_edit.jpg.

Land into property, taking over all the available Land for large-scale industrial farming in order to hoard People's subsistence as their own excess wealth. All this industrial farming is for export (to europe and north america) and not for local consumption. Thus, Natives who were self-sufficient before the armed conflict are quickly being reduced to wage labor status. As a direct result, their cultures are now at risk of being homogenized under the regime of globalization. And our Grandmother, the Land, has been transformed once again into property—owned by huge international conglomerate artificial persons called corporations. In that process, productive local farms were scraped flat to clear the Land for growing broccoli for the lucrative export industry. Indeed, I never saw broccoli served at any meal in guatemala.

One simple way to catalog this dramatic shift is to reflect on the different taste of Corn tortillas in the north and the south of Turtle Island. Anyone who has traveled south of the u.s. "border" in the past has experienced the spectacular difference in the taste of Corn in mexico, of course, but especially in central america: guatemala, honduras, el salvador with their high percentage of Native population. Tortillas taste different in guatemala! The bland cardboardy-taste of american grocery store tortillas is replaced by the shock of actual Corn flavor, tortillas that are handmade that same morning from ancient Corn rather than the mass-produced hybrids and packaging of the north. And in guatemala always in two colors: yellow Corn and especially the impeccable sweetness of blue Corn. One can still taste the difference in Indian Reservation communities that still plant their traditional seeds, but that quality simply cannot be replicated in industrial farming and modern factory production processes, especially when the seeds have been industrially bred for high-yield productivity rather than for actual quality. Our Grandmother has been traded out persistently with hybrid seed stock and highly processed production, all in order to maximize efficiency and thereby especially profits.

Beans, Squash, and Corn are a regular part of our family diet in Native communities here in the North as well. The Three Sisters are close Relatives; they are our Grandmothers. On our Osage Reservation, at least one family maintains that personal relationship by continuing to grow an

Osage traditional variety of Red Corn.[9] A Lenape colleague has, in his retirement, moved back to the traditional Lenape Lands of the Hudson Valley to grow the Three Sisters there, especially planting a special variety of Flint Corn. The Sisters traditionally grow together, as Squash provides shade for the ground to nurture the young emerging Corn and Beans and allows the ground to maintain its moisture; Corn in turn provides the upright for Beans as the vines wend their way up the stalks of Corn to support themselves. Thus, the Three Sisters nurture and support each other. Each uses different nutrients from the soil and then returns a different set of nutrients back to the soil to ensure the next harvest of the other two Sisters. And together, the Three Sisters form a protein that is a whole protein for sustaining human life.[10] Natives traditionally harvest them for food every fall to feed our families.

American Indian People care for these Three Sisters and are grateful for their existence every day. Many communities across Turtle Island have special annual ceremonies to honor these Relatives, like "Green Corn Ceremonies" at the time of the first harvests from the north to the southeast and across the continent. Indeed, part of our age-old agreement with the Sisters is showing our respect for them as close Relatives in ceremonial ways. Needless to say, that means we recognize the personhood of the Three Sisters and all our other Relatives that we consume for food. And even when we eat, we set some of the food aside to return to the *wanagi*, including the *wanagi* essence of the Sisters themselves, to include them in our mealtime and to show our gratitude. The Osage word *wanagi* here

---

9. The Osage Nation maintains a substantial farming operation in Pawhuska, Oklahoma, and the Red Corn family in particular have been instrumental in protecting and nurturing the planting and harvesting of Red Corn (*hába shutse*). I understand that Ryan Red Corn currently manages Red Corn Native Foods in Pawhuska, started decades ago by his grandfather, Raymond. A few years ago, I made regular trips from denver down to the San Juan Pueblo Reservation to stock up on Blue Corn. See, for example, carol clark, "Buffalo slaughter left lasting impact on Indigenous Peoples," emory news center, emory university, august 23, 2023.

10. See the Chickasaw Nation's write-up with their recipe for "Three Sisters stew": https://www.chickasaw.net/Our-Nation/Culture/Foods/Three-Sisters-Stew.aspx#:~:text=The%20Three%20Sisters%20is%20a,each%20other%20as%20they%20thrive.

refers to the spiritual essence of any person (needless to say, both human and other-than-human persons). That essence survives the person's physical body and continues life in another world, the *wanagi* world. Our food offerings maintain our relationships with Relatives in that *wanagi* world.

Because of the radical compromise Osages have made over the years under historical colonialist pressures, most Osages have stopped attending to the responsibility of making such a food offering. One of my own sisters tells me resolutely, "We don't do that anymore!" Yes, indeed. The colonizer and their missionaries worked very hard to destroy our ancestral connection with these Relatives, preferring that Osages learn to mimic the eurochristian devotion to some abstract and hierarchical male sky "god"[11] in lieu of remembering and relating to our actual, tangible Relatives that are constantly around us and share our territory with us. In one fell swoop, the collateral-egalitarian worldview of Native Peoples gets replaced with eurochristian hierarchy, including a hierarchy of being that envisions humans as occupying a higher status above the four-leggeds and above our Plant Relatives. She and he then become "it." Corn is no longer my Grandmother; rather, I am "its" master, free to do with "it" as I please. I buy "it," I own "it," and I eat "it" at will since I purchased "it" as property at the store. So, we have been co-opted into participating in creating disharmony and imbalance in the cosmos around us.

In spite of colonialism, however, many Indian People make the effort today to maintain those Relationships and to do our part to restore the Balance in the world around us. So, Natives remember to thank the Three Sisters, to thank the Buffalo, to thank any Relative that we use for food. In the same way, Natives also remember every drop of Water, our Grandfather, and every grain of Soil, our primordial Grandmother, who have nourished the Sisters so they can grow and provide us with food. We remember that by taking care of each other, these Three Sisters are taking care of all of us, as are Grandmother *mo^{n}zho^{n} iko*, the Land, and Grandfather Water, *ni itsiko*.

11. See tinker 2013, 167–179. Now online at: https://s3.amazonaws.com/iliff-edu/wp-content/uploads/2018/06/18155740/Tinker-Why-I-Do-Not-Believe-in-a-Creator-Conversations-on-Creation-Land-Justice-and-Life-Together.pdf.

On the one hand, living this way is hard work. Native people know from generations of experience that there is real physical, emotional, and spiritual effort in making a sincere and thoughtful offering prior to procuring any nutritional source. Going into a store and just buying "stuff" is so much easier. When we do that, however, we contribute directly to a much more radical disruption of cosmic Balance. Both our lives and the lives of our Plant and Animal Relatives are both devalued in that process. Our traditional ways are healthier, more sustainable, and balanced, and they enable us to maintain our relationships with these important Relatives in a spirit of gratitude.

It's early november as I finish writing, but I know that in three weeks many american participants from our Food Fight conference will be planning family feasts and reunions on that day most americans call thanksgiving and which many Natives with a sense of irony refer to as *thankstaking day*. Natives remember the loss of Land (and particularly our personal relationship with the Grandmother) and the colonizer principles of extraction, resource development, and commodification that have proven to be so destructive of our own communities and of our close Relatives who have become resource "things" to be developed for financial gain. Natives remember their eurochristian relatives as "takers" and notice that this same proclivity for taking continues in the colonizers' industrial extractive assaults across Turtle Island.

Of course, at this time of year we only need visualize the large pile of Turkeys stacked in an open freezer in every supermarket, walmart, or costco, usually laced with antibiotics and other supplemental chemical additives. Indeed, the more "clean" the turkeys, the more humane the farm, and the less they are chemically treated, the more expensive they become! Think organic, free-range, an so on; then notice how the prices go up from a dollar-twenty per pound to four and five dollars and even higher per pound. We can begin to see that the problem is systemic. Poor people are doomed to eat the least healthy foods produced by industrial farming and the most heavily processed foods that can be bought cheaply and eaten without expensive preparation. The same economic realities determine modern beef farming: Feedlot operations where cattle are imprisoned and fed processed corn-slop nonstop so they can develop high levels of meat tenderizing fat. From birth to slaughterhouse they never see a blade of grass.[12] Sure, free-range, grass-fed beef is available as an alternative, but only for those wealthy enough to buy it.

Until the colonial invasion of our Land, American Indians never had a single day each year for expressing gratitude. Rather, Natives walk the Earth with a spirit of gratitude with each step, every day, thankful for all Life in our world. We never expressed this gratitude to some abstract, hierarchical being, but rather we express gratitude directly to each of our Relations. Indeed, walking monzhon, Grandmother, the Earth with a spirit of gratitude at all times is fundamental to our Native worldview. In spite of 531 years of eurochristian colonialism and domination we continue to show our thankfulness. For American Indians, we live each day remembering all our Relatives and thanking them—Corn, Beans, Squash, the Water, the Earth herself, the Tree people and the Mountains, the Deer, the Buffalo, the Rivers.

This gratitude is important even as colonialist industry takes over so much of Grandmother and threatens the lives of all our Relatives. Salmon are threatened today by industrial projects that dam the Rivers used by those Relatives for spawning and regeneration each year. Mega corporations like georgia-pacific clear-cut forests, destroying the natural animal habitat and causing topsoil runoff into those same Rivers, polluting them beyond Salmon survival. Others are still cutting ancient and pristine Cedar or douglas Fir forests, depriving Native communities of yet other important Relatives.[13] Buffalo Relatives were nearly killed to extinction, and even today they only live on reservations set aside to contain them: Buffalo ranches and preserves that are carefully contained to keep beef cattle safe from infestation. Yet, we are grateful that our Buffalo siblings have continued to survive, sometimes even on our own reservations.

There is no contradiction that we consume our close Relatives and harvest others for clothing or housing needs in order to survive. Indeed, there

---

12. Note the important volume by poulan 2006.

13. Leyland cecco, "Photography campaign shows the grim aftermath of logging in canada's fragile forests," *the guardian* (2-12-2020): https://www.theguardian.com/world/2020/dec/02/canada-forests-clearcutting-ecosystem. And see the important chapter on old growth douglas fir in the northwest in kimmerer 2013, 341ff.

are stories in every community of how Corn, for instance, decided to give herself to humans for our sustenance.[14] Corn is also important as a Medicine: for instance, the Corn tassels can be steeped as a medicinal tea. Or how the four-leggeds decided in the long ago to let humans use some of themselves for food and shelter. At the same time, we humans dare never become disconnected from these close Relations as "takers," treating them as mere resources. Our goal is always to maintain Balance in the world around us, to live in Balance with all our Relations even as we necessarily disrupt the cosmic Balance of the universe whenever we eat. And that means we need to have explicit and trusted ways to correct that imbalance, to restore Balance, continually. That is our human responsibility back to our Relatives in the world around us. And there are clear protocols that call for ceremony to mark each of our Relatives as sacred that are intended to help us maintain Balance. Only then are we free to eat.

To understand the wholeness of Native relationships in the Americas, we could note a Haudenosaunee thanksgiving ceremony, a ceremony that takes considerable time to accomplish. In other words, the ceremony is completely contradictory to the modern commodified culture of convenience where "time is money." The thanksgiving address includes formal addresses to each of the Peoples of the world. In separate addresses within the whole, these persons, named personally and explicitly, include the Earth Mother, the Waters, Lakes and Rivers, the Fish, the Food Plants, the Medicine Herbs, the Animals, the Trees, the Birds, the Four Winds, the Thunderers, the Sun, Grandmother Moon, and the Stars, among others.[15] At stake in the addresses is the human responsibility to contribute to the harmony and Balance of the world around us—rather than the eurochristian sense of privilege or ownership that reduces the natural world to merely a bundle of potential resources to be taken, extracted.

For the eurochristian colonizer all these Relatives had necessarily to be converted, along with the Land itself, into reified objects or things and

---

14. See the now outdated tink tinker essay: "christology and colonialism: jesus, Corn Mother, and conquest," 2008, 84–111.

15. "Haudenosaunee thanksgiving address: greetings to the natural world," Mohawk version, 1993: https://americanindian.si.edu/environment/pdf/01_02_Thanksgiving_Address.pdf.

ultimately into property or potential property just waiting to be subdued (along with all of nature) by the arrogance of eurochristian ingenuity and labor. And for the eurochristian, profit and prosperity, the abstraction of money and wealth, become evidence of the righteousness of property ownership. The loss of the Natives' relationship with Land/the Earth becomes the steep price of conversion to the eurochristian colonialist way of thinking and living—to their worldview of the commodification and thingification of all our Relatives, serving in a hierarchy to satisfy the highest good of human beings and especially serving to enrich the richest humans.

So, the Land has become property now, and you will look in vain to find Beans or Squash growing with the corn as you drive through nebraska or iowa. Just endless fields of mass-produced hybrid corn, genetically redesigned for the market and for production quantity. You'll see huge and very expensive machinery being used to reap this harvest. No ceremony at all; just plenty of off-road diesel fuel pumping its smoke into what used to be pristine air. Wheat? Sure, amber fields of grain, but no people anywhere. Just barely visible inside his enclosed air-conditioned cab is the lone operator driving a five-hundred-thousand-dollar combine-machine to cut wheat in as many fields as he can in a few days before moving further north for the next harvest. Even this operator is a wage-laborer with little personal investment and no personal relationship with what he is harvesting. And at harvest time, he will work his way north with others in his laborer crew from texas all the way to canada, calling none of those places home. That is the efficiency it takes to have corn-fed beef or a box of wheaties on the kitchen table. Factory farming. And industrial eating.

This eurochristian proclivity to thingify our Relatives has been persistently globalized today. Now, we have saudi arabian industrial agricultural corporations leasing Land—and its Water—in the arizona desert to grow alfalfa to feed cattle back in saudi arabia to bolster their own growing industrialized beef addiction.[16] While eurochristians in arizona are crying

16. Isaac stanley-becker, joshua partlow and yonne wingett sanchez, "How a saudi firm tapped a gusher of Water in drought-stricken arizona," *washington post*, july 16, 2023; and ben tracy, "Saudi company draws unlimited arizona ground water to grow alfalfa amid drought," *cbs mornings*, april 20, 2023.

foul and insisting on government intervention to deny saudi access to what they declare is an "american" resource, no one is paying attention to what this industrial use of Water does to Native communities in arizona or the disrespect industrialization shows to *ni itsiko*, Grandfather Water, himself.[17] Did I say "himself"? They would systemically and automatically refer to him as "it," a thing to be extracted and monetized for profit. "It" is a necessity for life whose monetary value increases in a desert environment like arizona.

A couple of years ago, I made a very short video (under three minutes) for denver schools' "Native American culture and education" department titled, "The Three Sisters."[18] While this was vetted as an american "thanksgiving" teaching tool (aka, thankstaking day) for young Native kids, it was much more about the chasm of worldview difference that gapes between American Indians and eurochristian peoples. Corn, Beans, and Squash are in a close experiential relationship with Indian Peoples as our Grandmothers, who long ago offered themselves as sustenance for their human relatives to keep us alive and healthy. As a result, these relatives were held in high regard and always handled by humans with utter respect. Humans use ceremony whenever they plant the seeds of these Grandmothers or harvest their fruits as a way of showing their respect. Likewise, Buffalo, Salmon, and Rice (i.e., american Rice! Called "wild" by eurochristians, just like the Indians, I suppose) are in this world of ongoing and devastating industrial extraction, from industrial farming to mining the Earth for resources. The Water (*ni itsiko* or *wazhazhe itsiko*, Grandfather Water) upon which Rice and other close Relatives of Native Peoples depend is today being threatened by one mining or pipeline operation after another, each of which can desecrate millions of ground Water gallons each day to successfully feed the bank accounts of the already rich in places like minneapolis, new york, zurich, sydney, or toronto. Here I should add that Water is one of our oldest Grandparents and calls on Native respect in the same way as these other Plant and Animal Relatives do.

17. Here it might be useful to remember that the Native vote in the 2020 election denied donald trump victory in this state.

18. *Three Sisters*, 2021, https://vimeo.com/644058549.

Instead of working for Balance in the world, Balance with all our Relatives around us, under the dominance of eurochristian colonialism, we have opted for a teleology of creating endless new wealth for the already very wealthy. But eventually, there will be no things left for them to buy. So, as nestle corporation recklessly bought up Water rights around American Indian communities in the u.s. and canada, the ceo of nestle said straight out more than a decade ago that (drinking) Water should be treated as a commodity just like any other. Maybe if we all drank less bottled water. . . . Yes, let's make it about "me," the eurochristian individual, and not about corporate greed. That way we can all recycle our plastic bottles and feel good as our Grandmother, the Land, finds new ways to resist human trashing and to repeatedly signal the downturn of human dominance.

Avoiding "it" and "thing" in speaking english: To help our non-Native relatives have a better sense of this Native understanding relationship I want to call on these relatives to try a very simple but nearly impossible exercise. Try to eradicate from your speech all usages of the eurochristian words "it" and "thing" as you speak this colonial language called english. Robin Wall Kimmerer makes an analogous point in *Braiding Sweetgrass* (2013, 53), where she speaks of avoiding speaking of animals or plants as "things."[19] These two words are so ever-present in english usage that people speak them without giving them a second thought. The thingification of animals and plants is so deeply embedded in the eurochristian worldview that avoiding these words becomes a nearly impossible task. And we should add here that the words do not have easy counterparts in any Native language. One example might be to look at Osage pronouns (*ie wazhazhe*): *e*, *í*, and *íta* can be translated as he, her, and theirs; or they, him, and hers. No neuters! No things. No objects. Only persons. Perhaps we could add the word "resources" to our list of words to avoid. If we could finally think of our food as Relatives and not mere resources, perhaps we could begin to ensure that there was enough for everyone.

19. As a university biology professor, she continues to make the eurochristian distinction between humans and nature; yet as a Potawatomi woman, she acknowledges the personhood of all nonhuman Relatives that fall into the customary eurochristian category of nature.

With the invention of a money economy, which john locke explains is principally a means of storing wealth, we begin the process of commodification, thingification. That in turn assures that there is enough only for everyone who can afford to make the purchase, and corporations like nestle want to bottle as much Water as they can to ensure their own profits. After all, my Grandfather Water is today no more than a resource, a commodity to be conserved for selling piecemeal. The end result is not enough Water for many communities to thrive, both for drinking and for nurturing plant growth. And to complete their industrial extraction process, nestle has managed to corner (i.e., purchase) wonderful fresh Water resources on and especially near dozens of American Indian reservations across Turtle Island, leaving those Native communities suffering from severe Water shortages—and that on top of mining and oil pipeline operations and their Water devastation.[20]

But as we convert Grandmother, the Land, into property, we are denied our traditional relationship with our Grandmother. Likewise, when we commodify Water, Indians are denied our traditional relationship with that Grandfather. And the world is knocked out of Balance. As we mess with Grandmother and mess with Grandfather, they find ways to resist. To defend themselves, they create droughts, intense weather patterns of heat and cold that make factory farming even more challenging.

Lo, the poor farmer today. Yet there are no more farmers; or at least there are precious few. That is, there are few family farms left on Turtle Island. The farmers mourned in the press as droughts continue are in reality just businessmen struggling to balance their checkbooks in order to hire the necessary wage labor to plant and harvest the "stuff" we buy in grocery stores or "stuff" used for slop-feeding in cattle-lots and for making corn-flake cereals sweetened with corn-syrup.

---

20 Hiroko tabuchi and blacki migliozzi, "'Monster fracks' are getting far bigger, and far thirstier: giant new oil and gas wells that require astonishing volumes of water to fracture bedrock are threatening america's fragile aquifers." *new york times*, September 25, 2023. Nationwide, in terms of fracking alone, we are told, "fracking has used up nearly 1.5 trillion gallons of water since 2011. That's how much tap water the entire state of texas uses in a year."

Is our situation even repairable anymore? Is real Balance yet possible? If that is not a real possibility at this late date, maybe that is ok. As my elders explained forty or fifty years ago, Grandmother will survive—even with all the scars of reckless human striving for more and more hoarded wealth. "It might take another million years," the elders told us, "but Grandmother will heal—once she is finally rid of this virus called humans." Our choice now is either to relearn living in Balance and with respect for our nonhuman Relatives, or to accept our fate as a species dying off from self-inflicted wounds.

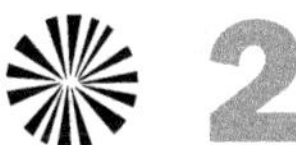 2

Sugar
The Bitter Aftertaste of Global Oppression

Miguel A. De La Torre

Sugar sweetens our daily tea and coffee, providing the needed burst of energy with which we start each day. Sucrose makes our pastries and cakes sinfully delicious, bringing a delightful end to the blandest of meals. This sweet crystallized material is the foundational ingredient for the ultimate aphrodisiac—a box of chocolate bonbons given each Valentine Day by the thirsty paramour hoping for reciprocal intimate sweets. Reserved once for royalty, aristocrats, and nobility, this formerly rare and costly substance can now be found in the barest cupboards of the world's poorest families. Once upon a time, our primate ancestors would satisfy their sweet tooth by furtively appropriating the sticky syrupy substance found in beehives. Honey, an animal product, has been known and consumed since early human evolution. Sugar, on the other hand, is an organic chemical from the carbohydrate family, a vegetable product extracted from plants through ingenious technical advances developed and slowly spread globally throughout human history, which has witnessed widespread usage only in the past two centuries. The two primary plants from which sugar is extracted are (1) the sugar cane, which has been the primary source of sucrose and is the focus of this chapter, and (2) the sugar beet, which was not economically viable until the mid-1800s. Today, we find it in almost everything we eat, causing havoc to our health. But it was not always so—for most of human history, sugar was not part of the daily diet.

Sugar has become so normalized in our daily diets that most of us fail to connect the blood-drenched history sugar production has caused. Probably no other food substance has caused more deaths due to its consumption, enslaved more people in its production, instigated the greatest forced migration ever known, created the greatest loss of biodiversity on the planet through the decimation of millions of plants and animals, or damaged more of the ecology in its cultivation. This sweet addictive substance is responsible for the ascent of empires and the descent of humanity. For sugar to become common, colonies were set up and civilizations exterminated, while the most brutal genocidal enslavement ever known was established throughout the Caribbean, decimating populations from the Americas, from Africa, and from Asia. It could even be argued that the modern concept of racism was sugar's firstborn, a necessary societal invention that facilitated its production. How then can something so sweet be so bitter?

SUGAR'S BIRTH

The birth of sugar is believed to have occurred on the island of New Guinea, located at the far end of today's Indonesian archipelago, around 8000 BCE (Mintz 1986, 19). From Indonesia, the sugar cane traveled to the Philippines, China, and India, where it was hybridized with other species. References to sugarcane can be found in Vedic-period hymns that date as far back as 1500 BCE. Eventually, someone in India discovered that if the sugar cane is boiled in a metal pan, along with some sort of alkali, sweet crystals would form. At first, sugar was prized for its supposed medicinal qualities. Gautama Buddha declared that it was not a sin for a sick person to ask for sugar. By the time Mahāyāna Buddhism was introduced in China, the Buddha was frequently referred to as "King of sugarcane" and/or "born of sugarcane" (Needham 1996, 61), while in China, sugar was used for many purposes, including as an aphrodisiac.

Eventually, sugar made its way to the Mediterranean basin, reaching Persia as an Indian hybrid, even making an appearance in the Hebrew Bible (Isaiah 6:20). The first European encounter with sugarcanes probably occurred during the conquests of Alexander the Great. By around 600 CE, there is evidence that Nestorian Christians were making sugar in Persia. The institutionalization of a *Pax Arabica* in the seventh century caused by the spread of Islam facilitated sugar's safe travel as commerce. In effect, sugar followed the Qur'an. The ability to securely transport sugar as a commodity provided an impetus to establish sugar manufacturing. By 700 CE, sugar could be found all along the Mediterranean. The Moorish conquest of the southern coast of Spain in 711 CE introduced sugar to Europe as it made its way as far north as Valencia. By 966 CE, the Republic of Venice was building warehouses to export sugar to Central Europe, the Black Sea, and Slavic countries. Along with spices and silk, the sugar trade was foundational in developing Venice's wealth.

By the dawn of the first millennium, the first Christian European Crusaders invaded Muslim territory, unleashing barbaric bloodletting. Many fought off starvation by chewing on the cane and surviving off the sap (Mintz 1986, 28). As these Crusaders returned from the so-called Holy Land, they spread throughout Western Europe the marvels of the sugarcane and the sweetness it yielded. With time, these Crusaders not only became controllers and supervisors of sugar production throughout the parts of the so-called Holy Land, which they conquered, they also helped transform Europe into a producer of sugar. With the fall of Syria in 1291, Christians retreating to Cyprus brought some sugarcane with them, prosperously transforming the island by making its wealth synonymous with sugar.

Soon sugar became a status symbol, a marker of social rank, a delicacy affordable only to the aristocracy. By the fourteenth century, the weight of sugar was equivalent in worth to the weight of silver (Toussaint-Samat [1987] 2009, 498). The rise of coffee, tea, and chocolate consumption propelled the need for cheaper and greater quantities of sugar. For sugar to be cheap, mass production was needed. For mass production to occur, slave labor was required. It was in Morocco and on the islands of Crete and Cyprus that the usage of enslaved people for the cultivation of sugar was first firmly established, creating an enduring link (Mintz 1986, 29).

The Portuguese in 1419 colonized an uninhabited island located some 1250 miles west of Northern Africa named Madeira. By the early 1420s, they began to settle the island, establishing sugar plantations as early as 1432. Not surprisingly, the African slave trade began shortly thereafter in 1441, when Portuguese sailor Antam Gonçalvez kidnapped a few Africans and condemned them to life-long servitude in the hopes of procuring the good graces of Prince Henry. It wasn't until January 8, 1455, that the usage of Africans as slaves for sugar production received religious justification through the Papal Bull *Romanus Pontilex* written by Pope Nicholas V. Confirming the papacy's claim to spiritual lordship of the whole world, the pope, as the world's arbitrator, provided Portugal with a monopoly over the African slave trade. The sugar produced on Madeira, although still considered a luxury spice, could be found throughout Europe by 1500, becoming the primary economic engine for the island. As early as the 1480s, sugarcane was being planted in the neighboring Canary Islands by the Spaniards and the island of São Tomé to the south by the Portuguese.

Africans were not the only ones being forced to work as sugar slaves. In 1493, during the height of the Inquisition, some two thousand Jewish children, ages two to ten, were sent to these islands to labor on the sugar plantations. Six hundred of them survived their first year of slavery; none survived beyond that first anniversary (Abbott 2009, 19). Over time, Africans became the sole human resource to produce sugar. Rather than being seen as an inhuman institution, the Spanish Church saw slavery as an opportunity to convert so-called African heathens to the true faith. More than simply a spiritual motivation, sugar was also profitable for the Mother Church. Dominicans, Franciscans, and Jesuits would also become involved with sugar cultivation in the so-called New World, meaning that they too would need slaves.

Sugarcane was first planted in the Americas on the island of Hispaniola (today's Dominican Republic) in 1493. By 1516, the first sugar made in Hispaniola was exported to Spain (Viola and Margolis 1991, 117). The cane grew so profusely that by 1518, eight sugar plantations manned by the indigenous Taíno population were in operation. It is believed that the magnificent royal palaces of Madrid and Toledo, built by Emperor Carlos V, were paid entirely from sugar profits (Toussaint-Samat [1987] 2009,

500). The Caribbean Basin was an economic construct whose *raison d'être* was the enrichment of the European homeland. Center-periphery relationships were established in which the empire's wealth building became dependent on the sugar produced upon these colonized lands.

SUGAR'S GENOCIDAL AFTERTASTE

The Taíno, the Caribbean island's first inhabitants, are believed to have emigrated from the tropical forests of Central and South America around 4190 BCE. For millennia they lived in relative peace. When a lost Cristoforo Colombo (known to English speakers as Christopher Columbus and to Spanish speakers as Cristóbal Colón) was discovered by the Taíno people, the world would forever be changed. During Colombo's second voyage of 1493, he brought sugarcane from Gomera in the Canary Islands, planting it on the island recently named Hispaniola. This singular act began the extinction of the Caribbean islands' Indigenous people and the genocidal subjugation of Indians on the mainland so that European empires could arise, a legacy that continues, to this day, to funnel most of the world's resources to wealthy Eurochristians.

At first, the indigenous Taíno were enslaved to mine gold and work the sugar plantation. Colombo was able to justify their enslavement due to a directive signed by King Fernando. The letter, written in Spanish to the Taíno, who neither spoke nor read the language, informed them that the pope gave their islands to the king and queen of Spain, and if the occupiers of the islands disputed this claim, they would be enslaved, their possessions seized, and their bodies harmed. The misery that would surely befall them if they refused to submit to Spanish authority would be their own fault for being obstinate and disobedient. This conquest led to women being raped, children being disembowelled, and men falling to the invaders' swords. Bartolomé de las Casas, an eyewitness to these events, wrote: "[The Spanish soldiers] would test their swords and their macho strength on captured Indians and place bets on slicing off heads or cutting of bodies in half with one blow." He recorded the death of seven thousand children within three months on the island to be named Cuba because their overworked mothers were so famished that they were unable to produce any milk to nurse them. Rather than seeing their babies suffer, they resorted to drowning them out of sheer desperation (1561, 94, 109–15).

What the sword did not fell, diseases decimated. The Spaniards brought with them influenza, measles, smallpox, whooping cough, tuberculosis, and other illnesses for which the native population had no immunity. The Taíno's way of life was further impacted when the Spaniards let loose upon the island vast droves of their livestock. Free from European diseases and local predators, these animals multiplied at an astonishing rate. Unfenced ranges led to freely roaming wildlife. Goats, horses, mules, donkeys, sheep, pigs, and domestic fowl thrived at the expense of Taíno agriculture. As these vast grazing herds destroyed crops, the food supply dwindled and famine ensued (De La Torre 2002, 6). This conquistador spirit that made its way to the so-called New World was fueled by a seven-hundred-year-old struggle to reclaim Spain and vanquish the Crescent by way of the Cross. As the last crusade against the Moors ended in 1492, a new, vaster campaign began in the Caribbean. Spaniards with little economic or political prospects in their own homeland would take their chances in the Americas. By coming to seize the land of others and work the original inhabitants to death to obtain glory and riches, they dreamt of returning to Spain with huge profits and mingling with royalty, nobility, and the gentry.

Spain's need for capital to finance its growing global ambitions meant that the new colonies in the Caribbean had to support the Spanish center and its quest for European dominance. Europeans, prior to the consolidation of power (1500), were politically insignificant when compared to the Ottoman Empire, China under the Ming dynasty, or northern India under the Mongol. But the so-called New World, with its enormous human and natural resources, provided the basis for transforming the marginalized Christian European principalities encircled by Islamic "infidels" [*sic*] into a world hegemonic power whose supremacy continues to be felt to this day. From the start of the European conquest, the Caribbean islands' enrichment of Europe, via Spain, occurred at their economic, political, and societal expense—a necessary outgrowth of having its economic surplus expropriated to generate economic development elsewhere.

The Spanish monarchs feared that conquistadors would become new powerful feudal lords. To prevent their accumulation of power, Queen Isabella and King Fernando passed laws forbidding the enslavement of the Indigenous population, which were routinely ignored. The political maneuvering of the monarchs to preserve their political space and avoid an emergence of feudalism in the new colonies was cloaked in piety. However, royal "sympathy" for the plight of the Indians could not overcome the demographic reality that Spain's population at the start of the 1500s was insufficient (due in part to the bubonic plagues of the previous century) for large-scale mining and crop cultivation in the Americas. Regardless of pietistic protest, someone was needed to cultivate the land and mine for minerals. As early as 1503, Queen Isabella wrote to her governor on Hispaniola expressing her desire to evangelize the Indians and the need for their labor. The Queen's will was satisfied through an economic structure developed known as the *encomiendas*, established in 1509 when Diego Colombo, governor of the Indies, was given royal authority to implement this system.

The word "*encomienda*" connotes entrusting a person to care for someone or something else. By removing the "ownership" of the Indigenous people from the Spanish settlers (whose increase in wealth could become a threat to the crown) and placing it in the hands of the ecclesiastical hierarchy, the crown continued to receive its revenue, the rising power of the conquistador was checked, the church obtained an opportunity to convert the so-called "savages," and the Indians supposedly benefitted from hearing the gospel and a set of rules designed to limit the degree of their exploitation for labor. This arrangement, which provided both free laborers and fertile soil, was more insidious than slavery, since the settler invested nothing in the worker. The conquistadors had no obligation or incentive to ensure their well-being.

Within a short time, Indigenous people throughout the Caribbean were working on sugar plantations. The first significant sugar planter was the surgeon Gonzalo de Velosa, who brought sugar experts from the Canary Islands to Hispaniola. By 1516, the king of Spain, Carlos V, was presented with six sugar loaves from *Nueva España* (New Spain). Yet it seems that whenever oppression reigns, resistance develops. The barbaric treatment of the Taíno led a young Dominican cleric, Bartolomé de las Casas, to dedicate his life to fighting for their humane treatment. For the remaining fifty years of his life, de las Casas devoted himself to the Indian plight, earning the title "Protector of the Indians." Unfortunately, he never challenged the legitimacy of Spain's colonial venture; rather, he attacked the abusive treatment of the Indigenous people at the hands of the Spanish colonizers. The so-called "Protector of the Indians" still had conquest on his mind, even though he hoped to accomplish this task without bloodshed. While he deserves applause for being among the first European voices to criticize the immoral stance of the conquistadors, he also deserves criticism for his tacit assumption that Spanish Christian society was superior to that of the Indigenous people. Although "saving" the Indian from bloodshed of the conquistador, de las Casas nonetheless contributed to their ethnocide, facilitating the task of the conquistadors in their colonial venture even though he wrote volumes against their brutality (Tinker 1993, 9–19).

The *encomienda* system finally ended in the eighteenth century—not due to any moral or Christian considerations, but because the economic need of Spain to strengthen its military meant that less of the tributes from the work of the Native people were left for the *criollos* (children of the conquistadors born in the Americas). Throughout this entire *encomienda* period, the Christian church was not only complicit with the genocide of the Indigenous population, but also profited from the slave-operated sugar plantations throughout the Caribbean. And while Catholic religious orders like the Franciscans, Jesuits, and Dominicans owned and operated sugar plantations, so too did Protestant groups like the Moravians, Anglicans, and Quakers.

SUGAR'S RACIST AFTERTASTE

Dogma extra ecclesiam nulla salus[1] provided a "positive" justification for *encomiendas*. Although Indian conversion to Christianity and civilization through conquest was normalized and the appropriation of their labor

---

1. "outside the church there is no salvation"

legitimized, their enslavement required philosophical, theological, and/or scientific justification. Aristotle's theory of "natural slaves" provided rationalization. He maintained that slavery was not an institution, but a category of humans. The Indians are not "slaves" because of the actions of the conquering Spaniards, or because of some divine will. Rather, they are "slaves" because the construction of the universe relegates some humans to the level of unthinking beasts in need of domestication to fulfill their natural calling of perpetual servitude. Juan Ginés de Sepúlveda, the era's main defender of the idea of cultural evolution, saw the difference between the Indigenous people and Europeans as one between barbarism and civilization. The Indian's sturdy bodies and "weak" brains displayed nature's intent for them to labor for the superiorly refined Europeans [sic].

The Indigenous population was being decimated by enslavement. Unlike other Latin American nations, Caribbean Indians were reduced to near extinction. A declining labor pool necessitated replacing this vanishing population; thus, Mayans from the Yucatan were first brought to Cuba to replace the Taíno. Being insufficient, peasants and rogue elements of the European population were brought as indentured servants to replace the decimated Indigenous labor pool, but this new alternative labor source proved ineffective. Brutal working conditions, epidemics, malnutrition, alcoholism, and brawls took a devastating toll. Besides, Europe's limited population of the 1500s was deficient in meeting the labor demand for the cultivation of the staple crop of sugar. An expendable work force was needed to make the large-scale production of sugar a reality, or else the Caribbean colonial enterprise would fail and European investors would be forced to declare financial ruin. If a slave population was not imported to the islands, the entire so-called "New World," from the European point of view, would be a financial bust.

As Indians became fewer in numbers, the so-called "Protector of the Indians" was approached by sugar planters requesting support to enslave Africans to replace Taínos. De las Casas agreed. After all, weren't African slaves already working in other sugar plantations within the Spanish realm? Weren't they more physically adept for the required hard labor? Although de las Casas would later repent in his complicity with establishing the African slave system, the damage was done. His carelessness facilitated the greatest coerced migration in human history, as some twelve million Africans were forced to leave their homes in crammed filthy ship holds. As many as two million would perish in transport in what has come to be known as the Middle Passage. The remaining nine to ten million were brought to the Americas, of which 25 percent were destined for the sugar plantations of the Caribbean (Viola and Margolis 1991, 121). The majority were men in the prime of their lives, facilitating an African brain and labor drain that caused economic underdevelopment for the continent.

Upon sugar the Caribbean islands' economies were created for the benefit of a few; because of sugar, liberation had to be denied to detriment of the many. Africans became the chosen race not because they were necessarily considered inferior (racism), but more importantly, because they were convenient (classism). Eric Williams states it best: "Slavery was not born of racism; rather racism was the consequence of slavery" (1942, 7). The expansion of sugar production throughout the Caribbean propelled the rapid growth of enslaved labor in the colonies and the rise of capitalism in the European motherland.

By the mid-1500s, sugar ceased being a luxury catered to the few and began to be enjoyed by the emerging middle class in Europe. As its popularity spread among the general population and production increased, prices for the sweetener began to fall from the equivalent of twenty-four US dollars a kilogram in 1350 to six US dollars in 1550. As prices fell, new growing markets developed (Macinnis 2002, 80–81). The demand for sugar spurred the expansion of large-scale sugar plantations as a means to the enrichment of European empires, thus satisfying the emergent sweet tooth of the European masses. But before the first sugarcane could be poked into the ground, thousands of acres surrounding the mill had to first be cleared, which was no small task. During the eighteenth century, islands throughout the Caribbean were literally set on fire to clear forests that stood in the way of sugarcane cultivation. For months, the smoke rising from these fires filled the sky and contributed to untold ecological devastation through the loss of the islands' biodiversity, as millions of plants and animals were decimated (Higman 2012, 63).

As important as sugar was in the making of desserts, its prominence subsided as bitter stimulants—coffee, tea, and chocolate—were introduced to Europe. By the 1700s, adding sugar to tea or coffee became so normative that even a poor farmer living in the outskirts of London could enjoy their drink sweetened. No longer a rarity, sugar became a mass-produced commodity (Mintz 1986, 46). Prior to the construction of factories that spurred the British Industrial Revolution, an assembly line process was already operating on the Caribbean sugar plantations. According to Eric Williams, these plantations "[Produced] tremendous wealth . . . from an unstable economy based on a single crop, which combined the vices of feudalism and capitalism with the virtues of neither" (1942, 13).

Here then is the colonial Caribbean equation, which was both classist and racist: without slavery there could not have been sugar. The volume of sugar production escalated in direct proportion to the increase of the enslaved population. Africans became the sugar plantations' newest labor pool and were preferred over indentured servants because the latter expected land at the conclusion of their employment contract. Besides, the enslaved were cheaper. The cost associated with hiring a white indentured servant for ten years was more expensive than buying an African who could be kept for the duration of their life. But while the labor by the enslaved might be cheap, it remained the largest single "investment" on the plantation, representing up to 33 percent of initial costs.

Planters moved toward slavery because it was beneficial to their bottom line; however, it also was beneficial for the colonial center. Slavery may have been necessary in the peripheral economy of the Caribbean, but it became crucial for the development of capitalism in the European center. Sugar's contribution to world trade helped create the conditions for Europe's own industrialization. As sugar prices continued to drop, the poor of the seventeenth century continued to increase consumption, making sugar a common dietary staple. It is estimated that in 1800, world sugar consumption (with almost all flowing to Europe) reached 245,000 tons. By 1890, it rose to over six million tons (Mintz 1986, 73). Sugar concealed the taste of food that was not necessarily fresh—specifically meat—it added flavor to flavorless food, and it was used as a preservative, especially with fruit. But the real importance of addictive sugar-saturated meals was that it helped energize the proletariat while satisfying their hunger pangs, which in turn allowed them to fuel the Industrial Revolution.

Enslaving Africans gave birth to a transport trade. Two triangular trading patterns were established in the 1600s and matured by the 1700s. The first and more profitable triangle consisted of European finished goods being traded for Africans who were taken to the Americas, specifically the Caribbean islands, where they were then exchanged for sugar, molasses, and rum for the European return trip. While the colonies provided the metropolis with raw material, they received from the metropolis finished goods, that is, refined sugar, tools, clothes, and machinery. This trade in human Black flesh fueled the European Industrial Revolution, providing capital for factory building and demand for finish manufactured goods and ornaments that could be traded for captured Africans. The wheels of the Industrial Revolution were greased with African blood. Profits from the trade were also able to fuel European wars for dominance and further colonial ventures. The trading of finished goods (bolstered by a new postmedieval economic theory known as mercantilism) benefited metropolises at the expense of the colonies, which remained economically dependent upon the metropolis. The rise of mercantilism meant the rise of slavery. Its eventual demise would also lead to the demise of slavery.

The second triangle brought New England dried cod and rum to Africa, slaves from Africa to the Caribbean islands, and molasses back to New England, where it was converted to rum. Additionally, livestock and foodstuffs were traded with the Caribbean islands for sugar and molasses, leaving North America with a tidy profit that was then used to purchase European, mainly English, finished manufactured goods. Trade with the sugar colonies was the major cause of the prosperity and development of New England and the Middle Colonies (Williams 1942, 108). Unfortunately for the British Empire, this second triangle conflicted with the mercantilist goals of the first triangle. This might explain the 1764 Sugar Act aimed at ending the trade in sugar and molasses from the non-British Indies. Eventually, an economic rupture between the British Empire and its thirteen colonies developed. It could be argued that Caribbean sugar, not the tea thrown overboard during the Boston Tea Party, was the main cause for the North American colonies declaring their independence from the British Empire.

The demand for sugar and the development of these trade routes triggered a demographic revolution as Africans were brought to the islands to work at the emerging sugar plantations. These sweat-soaked Africans worked an eighteen-hour day and a six-day week. Most planters, seeking to minimize costs, did not provide proper nutrition and care. Although slave laws required a daily supplement of six to eight plantains or an equal amount of starchy tubers, along with eight ounces of meat or fish and four ounces of rice or flour, in reality, the slave was fortunate if they received two meals: a breakfast of *tasajo* (a Cuban meal of shredded salted dried beef) and a dinner of plantains and corn or a sweet potato potage. Hungry slaves who dared to chew on a piece of sugar cane while working risked being whipped, beaten, or having their teeth knocked out to prevent them from ever chewing on sugar canes again (Abbott 2009, 106).

Unlike US slave plantations, which required fewer Africans to pick cotton and where the average plantation housed few families, sugar plantations required armies of mostly males, numbering in the hundreds. They were kept in *barracoons*, a wooden or cement dirt-floored barrack. The latrine was usually the *barracoon*'s corner. Swarms of flies, fleas, and ticks, coupled with a lack of ventilation, created an incubator for diseases. The enslaved were locked in and overseen by watchmen, lest they attempted escape (Montejo 1968, 58–59). Not surprisingly, death of the enslaved exceeded births, which necessitated new acquisitions. But why then, if slaves represented the major portion of a typically modest Cuban sugar plantation (approximately 33 percent of its value, compared to 17 percent for land, 6 percent for the mill, and 9 percent for the boiling house), were they not better cared for? It was considered more cost effective to work a slave to death and to purchase a new one than to expend the resources needed for adequate slave health care or to raise a slave from infancy. Bahian sugar planters in the mid-1700s calculated that enslaved laborers would make up their purchase price in three and a half years (Abbott 2009, 113, 156). Not surprisingly, life expectancy for an African after arriving in Cuba was seven years (Abbott 2009, 113, 156). Many, as a sign of protest, ended their lives by suicide—an attempt to "rob" the slaveholder of their "property" (46–47). Additionally, due to the belief in reincarnation within several African religious traditions, some held the conviction that death would allow them to be born free back in Africa (38). Entire books can be written on the sadistic treatment of Africans and how they were whipped, maimed, raped, and worked to death, but such explorations remain beyond the scope of this chapter.

Legal slavery quietly ended in the Caribbean when Cuba was forced to abolish slavery in 1886 by a Spanish royal decree. But its demise created new forms of oppressive structures. First, a new method of sugar production needed to be developed to compensate for the loss of free labor. Additionally, due to the devastation of the failed Ten Years' War for independence, there was a lack of funds to modernize mills and introduce newer complex refining techniques. A *colono* system was established where sugar growers rented land (like sharecroppers) from the mills. The *colono* brought their crops to the mills for refinement, and in the process, became dependent on the mill owners. With time, the *colonos* tended to be *criollos* while the mills became foreign (mainly US) owned (Whitney 2001, 189). Secondly, planters devised a new model of labor discipline that forced fieldhands under threat of hunger, supplanting the system of corporal punishment. The locks were removed from the slave quarters because hunger and the need for food kept the former enslaved confined. Some planters freed their enslaved prior to its abolition when they figured out it was cheaper to pay for their labor than their maintenance during enslavement. Hiring contracted labor rather than maintaining enslaved workers was at times 50 percent less costly; hence, the standard of living for the formerly enslaved fell in the 1870s once they were granted their liberty (Thomas 1971, 280). Under "freedom," the formerly enslaved were hired to work the sugar fields only during peak seasons and were left to fend for themselves during *el tiempo muerto* (the dead time—off peak seasons lasting from June through November). Slavery was replaced with the rural proletarization of Afrocubans. Nevertheless, during the busy season, planters struggled with labor shortages.

Even before slavery ended, sugar plantations began to search for new sources of human labor. They turned to Asia. Asian laborers were brought to the islands, specifically Cuba. Before the abolition of Cuban slavery and in anticipation to its eventual demise, Asians were procured as "indentured" servants to serve as an alternative to African slavery. Although Asians, mainly Chinese, were technically "free," their conditions were as horrific, if not worse than those working next to them who remained enslaved. Both systems, slavery and indentured servitude, were so compatible that they were able to operate side-by-side, thus meeting the labor needs of the sugar industry.

The opening of China to European penetration in the 1840s created a new potential source of labor as Asians were loaded at Macau for the deadly journey eastward. They were transported on the same ships previously used to transport Africans. As with African slave ships, an iron grating kept them separated from the quarterdeck, with cannons positioned to dominate the decks in the event of a rebellion. The first Asian laborers arrived in the Caribbean (Trinidad) in 1806. In 1847, the first 206 Asians were brought to Cuba, a number that increased to one hundred forty thousand during the next two decades, surging in 1939 to more than three hundred thousand. Just as a deadly Atlantic Middle Passage claimed the lives of Africans, so too was a Pacific Middle Passage created. As many as 20 percent of the Asian human cargo perished during the long voyage to the Americas. In some instances, almost half the Asian cargo perished in transport. When they arrived at the sugar plantation, they were held captive alongside enslaved Africans. For some, suicide was a better alternative than working on plantations. From 1850 to 1860, Cuba had the highest suicide rates in the world, 340 per million (compared to Spain's fifteen per million), of which 92.5 percent were among the Chinese (Guanche 1983, 319–20).

Asian laborers were technically not to be regarded as slaves; however, the distinction laid mainly in semantics. They usually arrived with an eight-year labor contract. Because they possessed no economic value after eight years, they tended to be treated worse than the enslaved. If an Asian indenture servant disobeyed "superiors," they were corrected with over twelve lashes and/or the stocks. They were usually paid four to ten pesos per month, although under a host of pretenses, substantial portions of their wage were extracted. Technically they were provided with clothes, food, medical treatment, and quarters. At the end of their contract, the laborer theoretically could become a tenant farmer or pay for a return passage to their native land. Few lived long enough to exercise either choice, for an estimated 75 percent died during their eight years of servitude (de Quesada 1925, 4–6). Those who survived usually lacked the funds to return to Asia. With no opportunities, many had little choice but to renew their contracts at the sugar plantations.

The result of this "free wage" system was so like slavery that, until abolition of the latter, both systems functioned alongside each other. The use of indentured servants did eventually help facilitate the transition from slavery to a wage system. Unfortunately, once African-based slavery was abolished, Chinese indentureship provided a large pool of unskilled laborers, thus undermining Black bargaining ability to negotiate fairer wages. Besides keeping wages depressed, resentment and interracial tension soon developed between Blacks and Chinese, preventing cooperation in joint resistance. In the final analysis, it didn't matter if the sugar plantation hunger for labor was met by Native, European, Africans, or Asians. It didn't matter if sugar was harvest by whites, reds, blacks, browns, yellows, or any combination thereof. All that sugar cared for was a people group to be exploited, leaving one to wonder how something so sweet had such a worldwide bitter aftertaste.

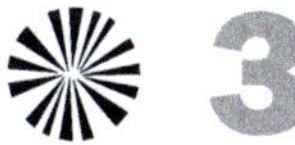 3

The Politics of Cultural Staples

When Indigenous Foods Are Misappropriated and Criminalized

Yvette R. Blair-Lavallais

I AM YVETTE BLAIR-LAVALLAIS, the sixth great-granddaughter of Matilda Berry, a mulatto woman, who traversed the systems of Black Codes and Jim Crow laws in the 1880s to make her way from Alabama to Texas with her adult daughter Mariah, a widow and mother of three sons. I bring you greetings from the Trinity River water basin where I reside on Comanche and Caddo Land. As a public theologian who studies the intersections of faith, food insecurity, gentrification, and displacement of Black, Brown, and Indigenous peoples, I am concerned with how we cultivate a food theology that disrupts and dismantles the weaponization of food, the misappropriation of cultural foods, and the systemic structures that racialize "cheap food" as a term of institutionalized violence. This theology, I contend, must also explore the relationship to, and be centered in, the context of food injustice.

The biblical text that will serve as the basis for the grounding of this discussion is found in Genesis 1:29. In God's economy, there is no hierarchy of foods (upscale versus cheap) nor is there a food desert. Instead, there is flourishing and continuous replenishing of food. Food desert is antithetical to the gospel of a Brown Christ, a God who is always on the side of the oppressed and who spoke this declaration in Genesis 1:29: "*Then God said, I now give to you all the plants on the earth that yield seeds and all the trees whose fruit produces its seeds within it. These will be yours for food.*" The problem is that *yours* has been contextualized to an *us* and *them* system in the framework of patriarchy and whiteness. The weaponization of food has been used as a political tool to erase the history of a culture and people. While much can be said about the interlocking systems of food injustice and land theft against Black, Latinx and Indigenous peoples, the primary focus here is to look historically at the root causes of food injustice in the United States and interrogate the practices and policies in which these disparities are anchored. Further, the categorization of "right foods" versus "wrong foods," that is, to declare indigenous foods as inferior and white colonists' foods as superior, adds to the complexities of how indigenous food and its history continue to be politicized in this country (Earle 2012, 3).

In the words of Winona LaDuke, a member of the Anishinaabeg Nation, "Food has a culture. It has a history. It has a story. It has relationships."[1] Each of these elements of food is compromised and interrupted when what we eat is weaponized and when it criminalizes one's culture. For the purposes of this chapter, Indigenous is understood as part of BIPOC, Black and Indigenous People of Color, which includes the cultures of Caribbean, Latinx, and African people. Because faith intersects with the work that I do, my research has led me to Samuel Argall, an English-born sailor who served as the deputy governor of Virginia during the two-year period of 1617 to 1619. History records him as beguiling and "nearly the author of the introduction of slavery in America."[2] Among the many dubious deeds for which he is remembered in history, including

---

1. Winona LaDuke. "Seeds of Our Ancestors. Seeds of Life." TEDxTC, March 4, 2012: https://www.youtube.com/watch?v=pHNlel72eQc.

2. John Esten Cooke, 1883. *Virginia: A History of the People*. Boston: Houghton, Mifflin. 111.

being a purveyor of Black enslaved bodies and "a human hawk in search of some prey to pounce on,"[3] there is one of particular interest and it all hinges on his instructions to the inhabitants of Jamestown to build a new church that was "50 foot long and twenty foot broad."[4] As a Black liberation theologian, I was curious to learn the historical significance of what has been described as a "*close-studded church built on a one-foot wide foundation of cobblestones.*"[5] This edifice, it turns out, was the site of a convening in 1620 where European colonizers gathered in the choir stand and legislated the theft of food from Native Americans. White settlers engaged in colonization of a people who were already here in America, encroached upon their land, and legalized stealing Native American staples like maize, squash, and beans. There was one other climactic moment that precipitated and set in motion four centuries of food injustice, what I will posit is food apartheid, a term coined by Karen Washington, a Black food justice activist, to draw attention to the "root causes of inequity in our food system based on race, class, and geography."[6] I understand food apartheid to constitute a system of structural racism that seeks to marginalize indigenous foodstuffs and interrupts people's access to food based on their race. It is perhaps one of the earliest forms of food injustice embedded in this country's foodways system. This disenfranchisement is prevalent in the iterations of how cultural foods, specific to Black, Latinx and Indigenous communities, are routinely misappropriated and criminalized by the dominant narrative of whiteness.

---

3. Cooke 1883, *Virginia*, 111.

4. *Jamestown Rediscovery: Historic Jamestown Website*: historicjamestowne.org/archaeology /map-of-discoveries/jamestown-churches/.

5. Virginia Company of London, Library of Congress, and Woodrow Wilson Collection. *The records of the Virginia Company of London*, edited by Susan M Washington Kingsbury: Govt. Print. Off., to 1935, 1906. Image. Retrieved from the Library of Congress, <www.loc.gov/item/06035006/>

6. Jo Walker, "'Food desert' vs. 'food apartheid': Which term best describes disparities in food access?," University of Michigan School for Environment and Sustainability, November 29, 2023, https://seas.umich.edu/news/food-desert-vs-food-apartheid-which-term-best-describes-disparities-food-access; Anna Brones. "Food Apartheid: The Root of the Problem with America's Grocery Stores" in *The Guardian*. May 15, 2018.

The American divide between who has access to food and who does not is a social, theological, and political injustice that dates to our colonial days. Food is political and has been since 1619, when European colonizers captured, forced, and enslaved Africans to come as disposable labor on the shores of the so-called New World. The destination of their new world, one that was mired in savage punishments and unimaginable pain—not the least of which was brutality and starvation—was on the threshold of a site with an oxymoronic name, Point Comfort, in what would eventually become Virginia.[7] Too often we have been presented with a sanitized version of history that omits this fact. To say that it was the apex of discomfort is to grossly misrepresent the agony, torture, and ungodly animus that was routinely and systematically exacted upon enslaved Africans.

When Africans were taken from their homeland—uprooted, kidnapped, and forcibly placed on slave ships—they left behind their families, their freedoms, and access to their cultural and diet-specific foods. Griots say that except for the few grains of rice and okra that enslaved Africans were able to hide in their braided hair, they endured the added trauma and anguish of relinquishing their bounty and abundance of healthy food. This was perhaps one of the earliest forms of politicizing and weaponizing food. Africans were not allowed to carry any of their cultural foods with them. Records show that in late August 1619, in a letter penned by John Rolfe, a Jamestown colonizer, to Sir Edwin Sandys, the architect of the so-called Great Charter that eventually led to the formation of Virginia's General Assembly, there is an account of what can arguably be the genesis of food injustice. Rolfe notes this about John Jope, the captain of an English privateer ship called the *White Lion* that transported enslaved Africans: "He brought not anything but some 20, and odd Negroes, which the Governor and Cape Marchant bought for victuals (whereof he was in great need as he pretended) at the best and easiest rates they could."[8] In befouled, cramped, and inhumane

---

7. David Smith, "Point Comfort: Where Slavery in America Began 400 Years Ago," *The Guardian*, August 14, 2019, https://www.theguardian.com/world/2019/aug/13/us-slavery-400-years-virginia-point-comfort.

8. "Twenty and Odd Negroes"; an Excerpt from a Letter from John Rolfe to Sir Edwin Sandys (1619/1620)," encyclopediavirginia.org/entries/twenty-and-odd-negroes-an-excerpt-from-a-letter-from-john-rolfe-to-sir-edwin-sandys-1619-1620/.

conditions, twenty plus Africans were pressed into an emerging food commerce system where they were traded for crops and supplies so that European enslavers could have access to food for their own survival and prosperity.

This meant that Africans were routinely traded for provisions such as rice, beans, yams, and other sustenance that sustained white settlers as they faced starvation as recorded in Virginia databases of slave trading voyages.[9] In particular, as Africans in America began planting and harvesting staples such as okra, watermelon, cowpeas, and black-eyed peas—foods indigenous to their homeland—these same foodstuffs were included in the trade negotiations where African men, women, and children were exchanged for provisions to meet the survival of their enslavers.[10] Not only were they exploited for their agricultural prowess in farming and forming this country's foodways and commerce system, but they were used as currency to buy food.[11] Since that time, as noted by food historian Michael W. Twitty,[12] these cultural-specific foods have been labeled as "slave food,"[13] an epithet that demoralizes and devalues not only the food, but also Black people. Black people had to improvise and use what was available and legally permissible just to maintain their diet. Throughout history we have witnessed iterations of legalized food insecurity and food injustice, designed to criminalize Black people. For instance, the Negro Act of 1740 enacted by the South Carolina General Assembly and included in the state's Slave Codes prohibited enslaved African people from growing their own food, earning money, assembling in groups, and learning to read.[14]

---

9. Lorena Walsh, Database of slave trading voyages to Virginia. "Transatlantic Slave Trade Voyages," Slavevoyages.org; retrieved September 12, 2023.

10. Daina Ramey Berry, *The Price for Their Pound of Flesh: The Value of the Enslaved, from Womb to Grave in Building a Nation* (Boston: Beacon Press, 2017), 7.

11. Jennifer Jensen Wallach, *Getting What We Need Ourselves: How Food Has Shaped African American Life* (Lanham, MD: Roman and Littlefield, 2019), 11.

12. Michael W. Twitty, *The Cooking Gene: A Journey Through African American Culinary History in the Old South* (Amistad Press, 2018), 4.

13. Wallach, *Getting What We Need*, 2019, 1–3.

14. American Legal History to the 1860s, Ch. 1.1. Primary Source: The South Carolina Slave Code, 1740, https://wisc.pb.unizin.org/ls261/chapter/ch 1-1-the-slave-code-of-south-carolina-1740/.

Food strategist Christopher Carter notes, "Our ancestors ate what we now call soul food in order to preserve their communities and promote their flourishing. Black people were forced to make the best out of the worst, and this improvisational ability is how we survived."[15] To be sure, it was survival food for both enslaved Africans and white enslavers. As America's foodways system grew and expanded, the food that once served as sustenance was dismissed by whites until it was repopularized and misappropriated. One of the most common meals that was once criminalized as "slave food" is Hoppin' John, a one-pot dish of rice and black-eyed peas enjoyed on New Year's Day as a way to welcome in new opportunities.[16]

The events of August 1619 were one of the earliest forms of a transactional sale in an emerging style of trading post where enslaved Africans were exchanged for food. Arguably, this was the genesis of a codified blueprint of ascribing economic power to food, a burgeoning system that became the standard at the expense of enslaved Africans. It was a repeated act where subjugating, disenfranchising, and depriving a group of people became the normative way of doing business. To intentionally swap people as a kind of currency for food and supplies was based on a reckless belief orchestrated by enslavers that white colonizers merited superiority over Black- and Brown-skinned people, all in the name of the gospel. After all, this arrival coincided with the convening of the First General Assembly, a patriarchal representation of twenty-two white males from every town, corporation, and plantation throughout the colony.

Their mission was to introduce "just laws for the happy guiding of the people,"[17] including economic arrangements, regulating moral offenses, and overseeing matters of religion and relations with the Powhatan Indians.

---

15. Christopher Carter, *The Spirit of Soul Food: Race, Faith and Food Justice*. (Chicago: University of Illinois, 2021), 2.

16. Olivia Ware Terenzio, "Feijoada and Hoppin' John: Dishing the African Diaspora in Brazil and the United States," *Southern Cultures* 25, no. 4 (Spring 2024), https://www.southerncultures.org/article/feijoada-and-hoppin-john/.

17. Susan Myra Kingsbury, ed., *Records of the Virginia Company, 1606–1626*, 3:98–109, The Thomas Jefferson Papers Series 8. Virginia Records Manuscripts. 1606–1737 (Washington, D.C.: Government Printing Office, 1906–1933).

In other words, they gave themselves permission to determine what was acceptable in their own sight. And they did it in the newly built church. It is here on the very floorboards of one of the earliest churches in what we now call America, where this scheme and immoral behavior of food injustice was birthed. This prideful self-imposed superiority is a belief in power and authority characterized by wanton violence, insolence, and outrage. That theology, cultivated in racism, helped to create the system of food apartheid. Karen Washington, a noted food justice activist and a founder of Black Urban Growers (BUGS), cultivated and uses this more accurate term of "food apartheid" rather than "food desert" because she says it is a system set up and maintained by human choices wherein some people are permitted to live in a community with access to a supermarket while others are not.[18] It is not a desert since that term implies a naturally occurring phenomenon where something has dried up. And the need for fresh food never dries up; moreover, grocery stores don't suddenly dry up either (Cummings 2019, 80–81).

This historical look gives us context to understand the root causes of food injustice and how it continues to be perpetuated today. I want to invite you to consider this fact through the lens of ecowomanist theology and racial justice. It is necessary for us to examine food theology and the ways in which Black, Brown, and Indigenous bodies historically have been starved, subjugated, and profaned by a Christian witness of whiteness that has misappropriated the gospel as made in the image of white supremacy—an ideological construct that has been promulgated and used to undergird a system of white privilege, one that has claimed land and food as their inherent right. In other words, white Christian food theology has been taught, preached, legalized, politically upheld, and endorsed, and as a result, it has manifested itself into the roots of our food system, including the way food is distributed and the way field laborers are treated. It is the reason that Black, Brown, and Indigenous peoples are categorically victimized in a system that criminalizes their cultural foods.

---

18. Karen Washington, "Frequently Asked Questions," https://www.karenthefarmer.com/faq-index.

As recently as 2018, a barista at a national coffee chain wrote a derogatory word on the coffee cup of a Latinx customer.[19] This word, a person who eats a particular legume, used to describe people of Mexican descent that associates them with a staple in their diet, is an epithet that stereotypes the Latinx community and the food that minoritized people eat. I prefer the term minoritized over minority because the latter suggests a ranking and devaluing of a person based on ethnicity or race. It is a cataloging or grouping of people of color that historically the United States has used to discredit and dismiss nonwhite people in a way that has been entrenched in oppression, discrimination, and racism. I don't believe that anyone is a minority in God's kindom (community of kinship). This racial slur emerged in the 1950s, and appeared in print in the late 1960s/early 1970s, as an intentional epithet against Mexican-Americans based on pinto beans being a staple in their diet.[20] Similarly, fry bread, a staple in Native American diets, has been "othered," and barbecue, traced back as a native food, has been referred to as "savage foods."[21] Barbecue and its variations of "barbacoa, barbikew, and barbicu referred not only to the smoked foods of American Indians, it also enacted Europeans' deep desire to see the food as barbarous and representing a kind of savage cooking."[22] This follows the same line of historically criminalizing Indigenous foods. "Ashcake and hoecake, baked in ashes on the blade of a hoe, were the staples of poor whites and, later, of black slaves, some of whom had known maize in Africa because of the slave traders, who imported the plant to feed slaves awaiting transport to the Americas."[23] Cornbread, akin to fry

---

19. David Williams, "Starbucks Faces More Racism Allegations after a Barista Wrote a Slur on a Latino Customer's Cup," CNN, May 17, 2018, https://www.cnn.com/2018/05/17/us/california-starbucks-racial-slur-trnd/index.html.

20. William Booth, "The Mouth of Mencia," *The Washington Post* (September 28, 2005), https://www.washingtonpost.com/wp-dyn/content/article/2005/09/27/AR2005092701875.html.

21. Andrew Warnes, *Savage Barbecue: Race, Culture and the Invention of Americas First Food* (University of Georgia, 2008), 3.

22. Warnes, *Savage Barbecue*, 6.

23. James Comer, *Cambridge World History of Food*, vol. 2, ed. Kenneth F. Kiple & Kriemhild Conee Ornelas. (Cambridge, United Kingdom: Cambridge University Press, 2000).

bread, was considered "poor people's food,"[24] though it was regularly consumed by whites with wealth. In an effort to distance white colonizers from eating the same foods as enslaved Africans, George Washington referred to black-eyed peas as cornfield peas instead, because the former was considered "slave food or "common food."[25]

While I was watching a cooking show on one of the cable networks, I found it perplexing and troublesome that the chef referred to salmon croquettes, a staple food popular in BIPOC diets, as "cheap food," but when sold in an upscale restaurant it changes tax brackets. The same core ingredients are being used, patted, and formed by hand into circular patties, yet the food is ascribed a hierarchical value based on where and how it is plated by the chef. This is an example of a cultural food that is often misappropriated where a culinary staple that is part of a BIPOC community is enjoyed as a privilege by people who have no connection or interest to the culture where the food originates. Similarly, hominy cakes, hot-water cornbread, and polenta cakes are all hand-patted cakes that are culturally specific foods that have been misappropriated by a white capitalist system. As Paloma Martinez-Cruz explores in her book, *Food Fight!: Millennial Mestizaje Meets the Culinary Marketplace*[26], misappropriation means sampling from another culture without establishing a relationship with that culture. At one time, these cultural staples were called "poor people's food" by the dominant white narrative, yet specifically the salmon croquettes made with salmon from a can are now being celebrated, whether made with fresh or canned salmon, and craved by upscale restaurateurs.[27] This is a nuanced layer of food apartheid that synthesizes the reality of the barriers and inequities that minoritized people face. Sean Sherman,

---

24. Joseph E. Holloway, 2006, "African crops and slave cuisine," California State university Northridge, Slave Rebellion website, ricediversity.org/out reach/educatorscorner/.../African Crops-and-Slave-Cuisine.doc (accessed January 2019).

25. Holloway, 2006.

26. Paloma Martinez-Cruz, *Food Fight!: Millennial Mestizaje Meets the Culinary Marketplace*. (Tucson: University of Arizona Press).

27. Yvette Blair-Lavallais, *Scrimpin' and Scrapin': The Hardships and Hustle of Women and Food Insecurity in Texas Through a Womanist Lens* (Charlotte: Arpege Books, 2022), 80.

an Oglala Lakota chef and founder of the Sioux Chef in Minneapolis, says, "The three sisters—corn, bean and squash—these diverse seeds are not only a direct connection to the past but a symbol of resistance to the destruction of our culture" (Sherman and Dooley 2017, 14). He employs a food theology of reclaiming these cultural staples and reconnecting a displaced people back to their land. This is how we confront the politicization of cultural foods.

To be sure, politics shows up in the layers of food injustice. Some fifty years ago, in 1974, Earl Butz, who served as the Secretary of Agriculture under Presidents Richard Nixon and Gerald Ford, declared that "food is a weapon. It is now one of the principal tools in our negotiating kit."[28] That is evident in this country's foodways system. Buffalo, a key protein source for Native Americans, were killed by colonizers as a way to punish First Peoples for not giving up their land. Records show that in the 1800s, white settlers proclaimed that "every buffalo dead is an Indian gone."[29] This portrays how deeply rooted and systemic food apartheid is in the United States. The lens of food apartheid gives us the language, context, and attention to the nuances of racism in our foodways systems—that is, the cultural, social, and economic practices related to the production, purchase, and consumption of food. Food apartheid also considers the behavior and implicit bias made about foodstuffs based on geography and ethnicity, and the ways that food is racialized. Because it elicits behavior of "othering" and the verbal abuse of using racial slurs, food apartheid in this way evokes violence.

Cynthia Moe-Lobeda suggests that "dismantling structural violence calls for identifying the cultural violence that nourishes it" (2020, 562). In other words, it calls for the oppressor to come to terms with their own culture of violence. This work of dismantling the systemic structures that cause food apartheid in predominately Black, Latinx, and Indigenous

---

28. "The food weapon and the strategic concept of food policy," in *The Ethics of Aid and Trade: U.S. Food Policy, Foreign Competition, and the Social Contract*, Cambridge Studies in Philosophy and Public Policy (Cambridge University Press, 1992), 20–40.

29. J. Weston Phippen, "Kill Every Buffalo You Can! Every Buffalo Dead Is an Indian Gone," *The Atlantic*, May 13, 2016.

communities could seemingly sound like a monumental task. Yet, this is communal work. What happened in 1619 and following was a disparate system planted with seeds of white privilege and rooted in racism. It was its own system of metaphorically genetically modifying an assertion of self-superiority, thereby othering and rendering a scale of inferiority to the enslaved bodies that were captured and to the Indigenous Native Americans bodies that would soon be forced off the land, mutilated, and killed, once more culturally castigating them in the name of God with all the underpinnings of a theology that was cultivated in hatred. This theology is not congruent with Jesus of Nazareth, a Palestinian Jew from the barrio born to a teenage mother. Instead, this evidences structural violence. Seth Holmes writes in *Fresh Fruit, Broken Bodies* that, "by structural violence, I mean the violence committed by configurations of social inequalities that in the end has injurious effects on bodies similar to the violence of a stabbing or shooting" (2013, 43).

According to the Native Agriculture & Food Systems Initiative, one in every four American Indian households is food insecure.[30] The US Department of Agriculture defines food insecurity as a household-level economic and social condition of limited or uncertain access to adequate food. What this also means as we explore this through a theological and ecowomanist lens, is that in many of our mainline denominations, there is an unmet impact that the gospel has yet to make on dismantling this economic and social unjust system of hunger. Again, I bring the church into this discussion because of its relevance as a meeting place in one of the most pivotal moments of 1619. As theologians, as members of the faith community, are we prepared to do the internal inventory of asking why the arc of justice is not yet bent toward our neighbors who are food insecure? Are we prepared to offer recompense about the ways in which the tempestuous origins of food apartheid contributed to the disparities that are still prevalent today? If we are merely preaching a gospel of abundance, many times in a community of food insecure neighbors, yet we are

30. Alicia Bell-Sheeter, "Food Sovereignty Assessment Tool, Native Agriculture and Food Systems Initiative, 2004, https://www.indigenousfoodsystems.org/sites/default/files/tools/FNDIFSATFinal.pdf.

not involved in changing the policies that have an impact on food insecurity, then is the proclaimed word returning void?

Within the theological framework of stewardship, have we been culpable in exacting a misappropriation of God's economy whereby we have engaged in a malfeasance of stewarding the crops of the land in a way that targets and favors white privilege and marginalizes members of the BIPOC community as inherently vulnerable? In what ways has the church been complicit in manufacturing and perpetuating food as a luxury, ensuring that the ones whom Jesus calls the least of these in Matthew's Gospel would always be disenfranchised in a food chain that was never meant to be hierarchical? These are the questions where we must engage in holy wrestling. Instead of preaching and constructing a framework of abundance, have we egregiously prescribed a lens that promotes a hermeneutic of lack, of oppression, of inadequate access to the bounty of food that God has provided? Have we so romanticized the miracle in the Gospel accounts of Jesus feeding five thousand men plus the uncounted thousands of women and children in a desert land, that we have failed to see that, like the disciples, the onus is ours to feed people healthy, culturally, and dietetically specific foods rather than send them home hungry? I argue that the disciples made a futile attempt to marginalize scores of people in the presence of Jesus and tried to get Christ, God incarnate, the word made flesh, to do the same. This, too, is structural violence. Isn't it something when we use food, in this case, the absence of, to weaponize, mistreat, and marginalize people? When we assign a ranking and devaluing of a person based on ethnicity, family background, and culture and attempt to discredit them as a minority, are we also consequently suggesting that they are undeserving of access to the abundance that is already in the Earth? There are no minorities in God's *kindom*. Intentionally I use kindom (with no g) to represent kinship and to remove the structure of power that is common in a monarchy where one is designated as king.

Has the church been the meeting place of legislators, delegates, and corporate giants who are members and who "read" about abundance, yet intentionally create a foodways system that sanctions and promotes the appearance of food scarcity, thereby writing and adopting policies that legislate the marginalization of BIPOC bodies because these decision-makers of power don't hear a gospel of bounty and access for *all* preached? How do we reconcile celebrating the eucharist, breaking bread and announcing that Jesus' body is given for all, when we willfully ignore the food injustices in our communities?

If I were to exegete and do the necessary theological investigation into what took place in the summer of 1619, I would see that delegates from Virginia's plantations convened in the church, the house of God, to plan and initiate the origins of food apartheid that has perpetually been the fork in the road that divides this country. It was at Jamestown, in the church, over a period of six days from July 30 to August 4, where delegates assembled in what history records as the first legislative assembly that governed the colonizers interactions with the Indigenous Native American Indians, for the primary purpose of creating policy that sanctioned, ordered, and constructed legal ways in which food—cultural staples—could lawfully be taken from them. They created, devised, and legalized a system that supported stealing food—in the church. This is food apartheid at the intersection of *the church*. Legislative assemblies are still happening as every five years the United States government reviews and renews the Farm Bill and makes decisions about agriculture and food policy. This means allocation of funds for food growth and distribution. The last iteration of the US Farm Bill was passed in 2018. The 2023 deadline for the next iteration passed as of the writing of this chapter, and there is a struggle to find bipartisan support on how food and access to food is legislated because food is sometimes red and sometimes blue. As a result, only a temporary extension through September 2024 was passed.[31] This is how food apartheid happens. It's a system. Food insecurity rises, the injustice deepens, and faith leaders continue to wrestle with cultivating a theology that resists these systemic injustices. Genesis 1:29 is a tenable place to begin building a theology that fortifies food security across the face of the whole earth. It also decriminalizes, depoliticizes, and reappropriates BIPOC foods. This theology is also the antidote to the political maneuvering of "othering" that leads to the erasure of a people and their cultural

31. Farm Aid, "Congress Passes Farm Bill Extension," November 16, 2023, https://www.farmaid.org/issues/farm-policy/the-latest-updates-on-the-2023-farm-bill/.

foods. Remember that food has a history and a relationship to a people, their culture, and their land. When you take away food, you take away history, relationship, culture, and connection to land.

Lawrence Davidson says this about cultural genocide: "it is the systematic erasure of the culture of Indigenous people subject to colonization."[32] He goes on to say "that the conquered land will no longer be popularly identified with the culture and traditions of those who were once native to it. Their culture will be replaced by the colonizer. Sometimes the colonizer will appropriate elements of the native culture as their own. This is theft, pure and simple."[33]

Finally, as efforts are being made to crystallize the approach to dismantling the systemic racist cogwheel in our foodways system, it is critical that we interrupt these systems that criminalize cultural staples. In our liturgies, prayers, petitions of the people, in our music and proclamation of the gospel, we must depoliticize foods of Black and Indigenous People of Color. We can no longer prioritize the benefactors of the system over those who are losing in the system. In other words, we cannot expect the beneficiaries of colonization to lead the way in dismantling four centennials of the criminalization food, in a system built by them, for them and made powerful because of them. In "Decolonizing Food Justice: Naming, Resisting and Researching Colonizing Forces in the Movement," researchers Katharine Bradley and Hank Herrera posit that "the cumulative effect of these manifestations of whiteness is structural racism and an unstated article of faith and nearly absolute certainty that the white way is the right way" (2016, 103).

This is the clarion call to the church, the faith community, to public theologians who bring their witness into the public sphere to address social injustices, with the help of Yahweh, the God who is on the side of the oppressed. Today is a good day to write a new narrative that honors the Native American, Mexican, and African American cultural foods that are the culinary foundation of this country.

---

32. Lawrence Davidson, "Food Theft as a Form of Cultural Genocide," *Counterpunch*, August 8, 2018.

33. Davidson, 2018.

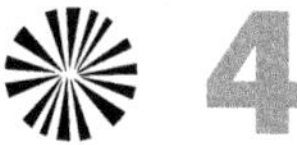 4

When Eating Fruits and Vegetables Hurts
Viewing Mexican, Latinx, and Indigenous Farm Labor as Racial Extractivism

Bernardo R. Vargas

PLANT-BASED DIETS CONTINUE TO GAIN POPULARITY in the United States, and Americans adopted vegan diets at a remarkable increase of 600 percent between 2014 and 2018 due to health and environmental concerns such as water use and greenhouse gas emissions from animal factory farming (Clem and Barthel 2021, 233–38).[1] However, consumers' increased consumption of fruits and vegetables intertwines with the exploitation of farmworkers, who play a vital role in growing, harvesting, collecting, and packaging produce. About half of the fruits and vegetables harvested in the United States require manual picking, which is necessary due to the meticulous attention to detail that machines cannot provide. This heavy reliance on manual labor underscores the crucial role played by farmwork-

1. Jennifer Bartashus and Gopal Srinivasan, "Plant-Based Foods Market to Hit $162 Billion in Next Decade, Projects Bloomberg Intelligence," *Bloomberg*, August 11, 2021.

ers, with 2.4 million agricultural workers in the United States (National Agricultural Statistics Service 2017).

In this chapter, I argue that the exploitation of farmworkers is better understood as racial extractivism, which emphasizes the centrality of race and colonialism in extractivist endeavors under neoliberalism, their influence on the economic framework, and social dynamics of production and consumption (Preston 2017, 356). I demonstrate this by presenting the enduring significance of the history of Mexican racialization in the United States and its rootedness in evolving colonial racial logics that become internalized into immigration laws and social ontologies. Focusing on Mexican racialization is salient as farmworkers, particularly those originating from México, have historically formed the largest group in the agricultural workforce of the United States (Gold et al. 2022, 4). By demonstrating the mechanisms of Mexican racialization, I reveal how those in power commodify Mexican bodies as a "resource" to be exploited. In addition, I display how these immigration laws are deeply rooted in colonial and white supremacy logic, which, when viewed from a racial extractivist perspective, allow these myriad injustices to appear as a continuation of the US colonial logic towards those racialized as Mexicans.

The plight of farmworkers remains one of the most salient environmental justice and environmental racism issues in the United States as it merges various entanglements between race, gender, immigration policies, environmental and climate justice, Indigeneity, and the legacy of colonialism and neoliberal capitalism. In addition to pesticide exposure, farmworkers experience a host of health and environmental precarity associated with climate change, such as exposure to wildfires and heat waves, as well as poor access to health care, barriers in language accessible to disaster information, infectious diseases, and invisibility from policymakers (M. Méndez et al. 2020, 51–52). These concerns are compounded by consumers' participation in the consumption of fruit and vegetable products, with an estimated 116.1 billion US dollars in profit for 2024, according to the 2024 Farm Sector Income Forecast.[2] Thus, farmworkers' rights ought to be paramount for

---

2. USDA Economic Research Service, https://www.ers.usda.gov/topics/farm-economy/farm-sector-income-finances/farm-sector-income-forecast/.

environmentalists and racial justice advocates, as an intersectional understanding of such precarity displays its pervasiveness through various spectrums (Crenshaw 1989).

RACIAL EXTRACTIVISM

Philosophical concepts prove valuable when implemented into historical case studies, as they illustrate abstract concepts through concrete cases and provide a better sense of the past and perhaps the present (Crasnow 2021, 78). When reflecting on the lineage of practices used by Canada's oil and gas industry, Jen Preston understands this extractivist history as racial extractivism. Preston's notion of racial extractivism emphasized how racialized communities and the environment become treated as "resources," subjecting people to a source of extraction for production and consumption within capitalist societies. Drawing on Cedric Robinson's work on racial capitalism, which posits that exploitation based on race and the accumulation of capital interact in a mutually reinforcing manner, Preston writes:

> Racial extractivism positions race and colonialism as central to extractivist projects under neoliberalism and underpins how these epistemologies are written into the economic structure and social relations of production and consumption. Racial extractivism acknowledges the multitude of ways in which colonial histories and reiterations of race-based epistemologies inform the discursive practices used by the oil and gas industry, for example, and by the Canadian white settler government in promoting and managing "resource extraction" (Preston 2017, 356; Robinson 2005, 2).

Preston's analysis of racial extractivism centers around two essential notions: extraction and racial capitalism. Extraction denotes a preliminary system of valuing someone or something in terms of financially profitable "resources" within capitalist systems. Political and social processes subject racialized individuals to harm that affects their communities and the environment. Preston argues that the transatlantic slave trade, driven by European empires' racial theories, was the largest extractivist project in history. Within this colonial project, Preston contends that extracting individuals or materials of value necessitated establishing a valuation system that intertwined colonialism, capitalism, labor markets, and the construction of the category of "human." This project relied on a deeply embedded logic of white supremacy and a construction of Blackness established within its colonies, which was used to justify the slave trade, influencing social and neoliberal economic structures (Preston 2017, 354–55).

A broader system of oppression sustains racial extractivism, which Preston identifies as racial capitalism, drawing from Cedric Robinson's seminal work *Black Marxism*. Robinson contends that capitalism not only necessitates an exploitable workforce to maximize profits, but capitalism particularly needs race. Robinson identifies what he calls "racialism" as the process of legitimizing and validating social structures as natural by reference to the "racial" characteristics of their components (Robinson 2005, 2). According to Robinson, the social hierarchy established on racial grounds existed before the emergence of capitalism but continues to shape the contemporary global system. This system's epistemologies are deeply embedded within neoliberal economic structures, legitimizing practices such as slavery, violence, colonialism, imperialism, and genocide (Preston 2017, 355).

As the historical analysis will reveal, the concept of being "Mexican" is intertwined with a social construct rooted in elementary eugenic ideas of "mixed blood," leading to the racialization of individuals into an intermediary category. This positioning within the white supremacy racial hierarchy placed individuals labeled as "Mexican" in a specific social imaginary, namely between racial categories of white, Black, and Indigenous. This construction of the "Mexican" social imaginary evolves, extending racialization to encompass other Latinx and Indigenous peoples beyond mere nationality. This racialization effectively excludes them from the privileges and rights associated with whiteness, as well as from conceptions of American identity, legality, and citizenship. "Whiteness" in this context denotes an analytical classification signifying the systemic benefits received by white individuals due to historical and ongoing discriminatory practices (Lipsitz 2007, 13). As argued by scholars such as Leong (2012, 2159–2160), whiteness operates as a form of property, determining access to protections, rights, and influence. Consequently, the failure to assimilate into whiteness serves as the mechanism for one's subordination.

Historically, labor extraction from México and Central America has been marked by "racialization," meaning the process by which human bodies are visually read, understood, and narrated using symbolic meaning and association (Omi and Winant 2015). Thus, the term "racialized" denotes groups that undergo this process, emphasizing the constructed nature of the category (Molina 2014). When thinking about racism, Linda Martín Alcoff asserts that, at times, ethnic categories in the United States, such as "Puerto Ricans" or "Mexicans," have racialized connotations, which is not the case for all ethnic terms, such as "French" or "Danish." She argues that some ethnic or cultural categories go beyond mere ethnic identification or skin color and extend into negative racist attributions such as innate natures, traits, or dispositions, similar to how a concept of race operates (Gracia 2007, 177). Terms such as "Mexican," "illegal," "immigrant," and "alien" can carry negative connotations associated with racial inferiority, violence, disease, and other racially charged ideas.

Racialization continues to be instituted in immigration laws, protecting the profit and affordability of consumers' fruits and vegetables while simultaneously placing farmworkers in dire living and working conditions. Through racial extractivism as an analytic, one can scrutinize how the process of racialization serves to justify the exploitation of individuals, essentially viewing them as mere "resources" for the accumulation of capital. Like the experiences of other racial groups, Mexican dehumanization originates from negative racial stereotypes, relegating them to a subhuman status or positioning them below a normative white standard, thus denying them equal protection, rights, and influence.

Adding to Preston's notion, in the case study of farmworkers, it is crucial to highlight the importance of labor as a fundamental aspect of the commodification of nonwhite people based on their racialization within racial extractivism. Two primary components of labor become assessed for value. The first aspect involves valuing labor as cheap: farmworkers are financially undercompensated, resulting in affordable fruits and vegetables. For instance, low wages for the physically exhausting work of harvesting fruits and vegetables enable the population of the United States to purchase them at low prices, which would inevitably rise if workers were fairly compensated (Calvin et al. 2022, 1, 18). The second aspect focuses on how racialized perceptions shape the evaluation of farmworkers' bodies and humanity, seeing their bodies primarily as tools for labor. This fundamental devaluation of their existence, with whiteness receiving greater value, leads to severe living conditions and environmental injustices. These two forms of valuation impact the affordability of agricultural produce and emphasize labor exploitation, which is particularly notable in México; both build on each other with pernicious consequences.

RACIALIZATION OF MEXICANS BEFORE THE BRACERO PROGRAM

To grasp the present challenges around immigration and food consumption, one must comprehend the historical impacts of US colonialism, particularly during the Mexican-American War of 1848, where the racialization of Mexicans becomes most apparent in the legal literature. The historical significance of the Bracero Program displays how racial extractivist logics defined the consumption of farmworker labor in the United States and continued the implementation of racialized laws that aim to recruit and displace Mexican farmworkers. White supremacist ideologies fueled the mistreatment, and harsh labor conditions experienced by Mexican workers represent one of the most perilous instances of violence against this ethnic group in the United States.

Within this historical context, it is salient to recall that the colonization of northern México by Anglos (and some Mexican citizens) primarily aimed to acquire land to support the enslavement of Africans for labor. Since México outlawed slavery in 1829, Mexicans soon came to be perceived as a threat to the enterprise of slavery and, thus, the economy of the United States (Ortiz 2018, 39–53; Molina 2014, 33). For example, in 1836, congressman and former president John Quincy Adams delivered a speech in the House of Representatives describing the United States' fear of the Second Seminole War and the soon-to-come independence of México, which would include the outlawing of slavery at the southern border. Adams proclaimed the following anti-Mexican ethos of the time, "Do not you, an Anglo-Saxon, slave-holding exterminator of Indians, from the bottom of your soul, hate the Mexican-Spaniard-Indian, emancipator of slaves, and abolisher of slavery? And do you think that your hatred is not with equal cordiality returned?" (Ortiz 2018, 43–44).

This quotation showcases a racial taxonomy: that of enslaved Africans, Indigenous people, a "hybrid" race (Mexicans), and Anglo-Saxons. This social ontology presents the Mexicans as both subhuman (sub-Anglo Saxon) and as an enemy due to their emancipatory values. The quotation also delineates the cleft between the colonial European superiority between Anglo-Saxons and Spaniards. To Anglo-Saxons, Mexicans contained the eugenic notions of "Spanish blood" and did not share the European privilege of whiteness and were, therefore, racially subordinate beings. The ethnicity of "Mexican" begins to be transformed into an "othering," functioning as a racial category, attached with the social meaning of a character to be despised by the highest officials of the neighboring empire. This racialization as subwhite and Mexican interference with the enslavement of Africans and the production of capital serves as a justification for the colonization of Northern México.

An additional fundamental justification for the colonization of northern México was the United States/Anglo's perception of the epistemic inability of the Mexican people to govern themselves. Secretary of State James Buchanan echoed the sentiments of many when questioning what actions should be taken concerning the statehood of Mexicans, "How should we govern the mongrel race which inhabits [the new territory]? Could we admit them to seats in our Senate and House of Representatives? Are they capable of Self-Government as States of this Confederacy?" (Gómez 2008, 42). This quotation displays a common colonial logic: those who do not meet the standards of white-European theologies and epistemologies due to how they are racialized and imagined to occupy an inferior epistemic status as "irrational" and politically "uncivilized." Mexicans were also familiar with this rhetoric, as expressed by Mexican legislators during some of the negotiations after the war, "The North Americans hate us, their orators deprecate us even in speeches in which they recognize the justice of our cause, and they consider us unable to form a single nation or society with them" (Gómez 2008, 44).

The idea of Mexicans' inability to govern themselves was deeply tied to the notions of Mexicans as "mixed," namely, part "Indian." Indigenous people were regarded late until the 1800s as "savage" and "uncivilized." Sylvia Wynter calls the "savage" classification the "savage Other," which functions from an understanding of humans (Man) as one who is rational and Christian (Hyatt et al. 1995, 35). Consequently, this colonial logic becomes applied to Mexicans' "mixed blood," justifying their colonization and lack of inclusion into seats of power. This inclusion of Indigenous "blood" would designate them as inferior to white racial imaginaries (Molina 2014, 35).

Thus, it is critical to note that the ethnicity of Mexicans operates beyond an identifying ethnic group or nation-state to that of a racial category with similar colonial and white supremacy logic to justify their colonization. Gómez argues that Mexicans disrupted the racial hierarchy in the United States by introducing a new racial category, as Mexicans did not fit into the Black or Indian racialization due to their European-Spanish ancestry, blurring the binary racial lines. Nevertheless, Mexicans' bodies carried the meaning of "savage" and "unruly," tied to racial imaginaries that did not allow them to partake in their European privileges.

As the border crossed northern Mexicans after the Mexican-American War, the Mexican people crossed new geographical boundaries and new geographies of racial logic. The moment Anglos set their gaze upon the Mexicans, they transformed them into a nonwhite, and most often, a subhuman other. The racialization of Mexicans continues to develop throughout the timeline as race never remains static, and it becomes embedded into the extraction of labor through its laws and perceptions of immigrant farmworkers until now

THE BRACERO PROGRAM

Initially established in response to the labor shortage during the Second World War, the Bracero Program, spanning from 1942 to 1964, led to approximately 4.5 million contracted workers entering the United States (Foley 2014, 126; Mize and Swords 2010, 3; Molina 2014, 112). During the Second World War, México and the US government established a series of three agreements known collectively as the Bracero Program, which resulted in one of the most extensive migrations from México to the United States. The Bracero Program shaped the current Mexican population in the United States and the contemporary United States' reliance on undocumented and contracted farmworkers. Although the two countries agreed on the Bracero Program to provide labor in exchange for wages, housing, and repatriations for Mexican workers, they repeatedly broke these promises from the program's inception. The International Executive Agreement 1949 required employers to sign an oath not to employ undocumented workers and to provide hospital and medical needs, yet farmers repeatedly violated this law (Foley 2014, 133–34). Farm owners' noncompliance with these laws would, at most, lead to the cancellation of their Bracero contracts, leading to border state employers quickly finding undocumented workers (Foley 2014, 134).

This new recurring pattern of the hiring of undocumented workers continues to emerge until the present. Farm owners' reliance on undocumented workers offers inexpensive labor and contributes significant financial profit (Molina 2014, 113). Farm owners consistently hired undocumented labor, justifying their decision by citing the perceived high cost of employing documented braceros. For instance, South Texas growers gained an additional five million dollars in profits during the Bracero Program, mainly stemming from the lower wages paid to undocumented workers (Foley 2014, 126). The consequences of this undocumented hiring were also minimal for employers in comparison to the poor wages, working conditions, abuses, and deportations that Mexican workers endured.

During the Bracero Program era, widespread anti-Mexican discrimination flourished, leading to heightened racial segregation laws like Texas-style Jim Crow. The Mexican government's response was to withhold workers from Texas between 1942 and 1947, fueling a surge in demand for undocumented laborers (Foley 2014, 27–28; Montejano 1987, 268). The Mexican government was hesitant to send Mexican laborers into the United States until the United States government guaranteed the rights of the guest laborers, which resulted in the second renewal of the Bracero Program of 1948. Due to the prevalence of discrimination, the Mexican government informed the braceros that it had obtained assurances that the United States would treat them with human dignity and that it would not subject them to social and economic discrimination due to their race, beliefs, color, or nationality (Foley 2014, 133). However, the renewal of the Bracero Program of 1948 failed to enact the promised guarantee of employer compliance for Bracero contracts and failed to stop the hiring of undocumented labor.

Stemming from México's complicity with colonization and racial logics, the Mexican government insisted that the braceros proved themselves worthy to their white-Anglo neighbors by maintaining their personal hygiene and obeying all laws and customs "in order to demonstrate that México is a civilized nation" and to avoid the humiliation of being denied admittance to public spaces, as Mexicans understood themselves to represent their traditions and their *raza*—race (Foley 2014, 133). Once more, the theme of race and epistemic incapacity to self-govern emerges, this time from the viewpoint of the Mexican government, where ideas and aspirations toward achieving a particular sense of "civilization" take on significance.

Even one hundred years after the Mexican-American War, coloniality remained palpable as the Mexican government conceived itself as being part of a different racial category (participating within colonial racial logics) and pursuing a notion of being "civilized," which in this case is tied to whiteness.[3] Here, we see how race-based epistemologies function on both sides of the border. The Anglo-Saxon's self-perception of racial superiority represented an entanglement of whiteness and citizenship rights. Meanwhile, Mexicans, perceiving themselves as a *raza*, relied on notions of "mestizaje" with its aim towards the attainment of whiteness and colonial logics of "civilization." Both sides bear and present the effects of colonization and the lingering coloniality that informed their political and social identity.

In the 1940s, the established ideas of racial inferiority to Anglo-Saxons began to influence agricultural and immigration laws and practices, exploiting those seen as outsiders. As racial extractivism centralized the role of race and colonialism within extractivist projects, one begins to see the interworking of how these racial epistemologies informed the laws and management of Mexican bodies as "resources" to be extracted for

3. Coloniality denotes enduring power structures that originated from colonialism but continue to influence culture, labor, interpersonal relationships, gender, and the generation of knowledge far beyond the narrow confines of colonial governance (Maldonado-Torres 2007, 243).

labor. Mexican labor here is used as a means to perpetuate more profit with minimal responsibility and consequences for those who hired undocumented labor or neglected the humanitarian standards agreed upon for documented labor. The colonized geography is now a recipient of labor extraction from México and rationalized by racial imaginaries and notions of Mexican people, which inform the immigration, social, and economic structure. Racialization entails the demarcation of boundaries within racial hierarchies and between those perceived as immigrants/aliens versus native Americans, delineating insiders and outsiders. This differentiation underpins notions of complete humanity versus denial, justifying disparate treatment, particularly pronounced in specific historical epochs.

REPATRIATION PROGRAMS

Concerns among Anglos persisted regarding undocumented workers, derogatorily referred to as "wetbacks," leading to the officially known 1954 Operation Wetback by the US Justice Department. The term "wetback" is a racialized term, as it propagated notions of "immigrant" and criminalization of undocumented entry, which was applied to both Mexican immigrants and Mexican Americans (Molina 2014, 113–14). The program was a massive military-style campaign that resulted in the deportation of 1.3 million Mexicans, including legal temporary immigrants and United States citizens of Mexican descent (Mize and Swords 2010, 25; Montejano 1987, 273). These deportations through buses and boats were cruel, resulting in the deaths of eighty-eight braceros due to heatstroke and harsh conditions (Mize and Swords, 2010). Operation Wetback also brought little to no responsibility to those who hired this undocumented labor (Mize and Swords 2010, 35; Hernández 2006, 440).

The expulsion of Mexicans was due to the compounding racialized fear of Mexicans. By 1954, México supplied the United States with approximately eight hundred thousand immigrant workers annually. The United States' pursuit of economic prosperity hinges on the regulated extraction of Mexicans, namely that of undocumented labor. The farmworker is, without a doubt, a substantive and essential means for producing various crops, providing cheap labor, large profits for producers, and, as a result, low consumer prices. The farmworker immigrants are extracted subjects for a dehumanized system of production, always at risk of becoming disposable. Their disposability manifests through a racialized threat of the nonwhite Other. Institutionalized laws and regulations heavily police and violently harm subjects. Operation Wetback was one of many subsequent governmental anti-immigratory acts to come, such as Operation Gatekeeper (California, 1994), Operation Hold-the-Line (Texas, 1994), and Operation Safeguard (Arizona, 1990) (Foley 2014, 123–24). In comparison, authorities minimally reprimand those who hire such labor and the consumers who benefit from it. It would not be until the Immigration Reform and Control Act of 1986 that employers, for the first time, were held accountable for hiring undocumented workers (Foley 2014, xxii–xxiii; Finch 1990, 251).

THE BIRTH OF H-2A VISAS AND THE CONTEMPORARY MIGRATION REGIME

After Operation Wetback, the US government had to address the high influx of undocumented workers, prompting the passage of the Immigration and Nationality Act of 1965 and the introduction of H-2 visas. In 1986, these visas would become the contemporary H-2A visas, which are temporary agricultural working permits with no paths to citizenship (Mize and Swords 2010, 34–39, 94). For farm owners to hire H-2A workers, they must demonstrate that there are not enough workers willing, qualified, and available to do the labor work in the United States.[4] Contrary to the common rhetoric of "illegals" taking US jobs, the low pay—ranging from eleven to sixteen dollars per hour in 2021—and harsh working conditions have actually led to a significant shortage of United States farmworkers, making it possible for farm owners to hire H-2A workers.[5] According to the FWD, a bipartisan political organization, as of 2019, 258,000 immigrant workers obtained temporary H2-A visas, constituting

4. "H-2A Temporary Agricultural Workers," U.S. Citizenship and Immigration Services Website: https://www.uscis.gov/working-in-the-united-states/temporary-workers/h-2a-temporary-agricultural-workers.

5. "Description of Chart: Adverse Effect Wage Rates (AEWR), 2021," United States Department of Agriculture: https://www.ers.usda.gov/webdocs/charts/86864/aewr2021_d.html?v=658.2.

only 4 percent of the workers required for total food production. Additionally, around 50 percent of farmworkers' jobs are held by unauthorized workers.[6] Between 2021 and 2022, 93 percent of those allotted H-2A visas went to México, with the rest going to South Africa, Jamaica, and Guatemala.[7]

In this neoliberal racial environment, the immigrant farmworker has not been bestowed citizenship, economic compensation, or the benefits of whiteness and continues to be perceived as an intruder, an undocumented alien. Financial demarcation based on racial division remains evident within the larger economic spectrum, with whites owning 98 percent of farmland and generating 98 percent of farm-related income and 97 percent of operation profit, while Latinxs primarily work as farmworkers (Horst and Marion 2019, 11). These statistics are significant as they highlight the racial and economic disparities among Latinx communities, which have persisted over many decades despite the historical legacy of discrimination, violence, and environmental racism.

Within the context of racial extractivism, which acknowledges the enduring impact of colonial ideologies, these labor extractivist projects transcend mere notions of raceless exploitation. Instead, they underscore the ongoing influence of colonial legacies on policies, economic structures, and opportunities for the most marginalized groups. This disproportionality is even greater for the 6 percent of agricultural workers who are Indigenous.[8] According to Michael Méndez et al. (2020), Indigenous farmworkers in California face dire socioeconomic circumstances, which places them in precarious circumstances. They point out that annual earnings for undocumented Indigenous communities generally fall within the

6. Andrew Moriarty, "Immigrant Farmworkers and America's Food Production—5 Things to Know," *FWD.us*, September 14, 2022, https://www.fwd.us/news/immigrant-farmworkers-and-americas-food-production-5-things-to-know/.

7. Philip Marin, "A Look at H-2A Growth and Reform in 2021 and 2022, "*Wilson Center*, January 3, 2022, https://www.wilsoncenter.org/article/look-h-2a-growth-and-reform-2021-and-2022.

8. "Indigenous Agricultural Workers Fact Sheet," National Center for Farmworker Health, December, 2021: https://www.ncfh.org/indigenous-agricultural-workers-fact-sheet.html.

range of $17,500 to $19,999. Among them, 40 percent lack medical insurance, and approximately one in five male farmworkers in California exhibit risk factors for chronic illnesses, including elevated serum cholesterol, hypertension, or obesity (2020, 53). Upon arriving in the United States due to displacement, many Indigenous people and other undocumented mestizos experience many difficulties, such as exposure to dangerous pesticides, disproportionate infection rates of diseases such as COVID-19, high rates of asthma among children, and polluted water (Carter-Pokras et al. 2007, 4).

Racialization and legal status determine how certain workers are exploited by the economic and political structures to the benefit of profit and whiteness. Racial epistemologies inform the laws that extract labor, namely undocumented labor, which can be better understood as "resource" extraction as it yields large profits with no path to citizenship and attainments to whiteness. To grasp the racial extractivist dynamics at play, one must examine how racialization occurs in space and how race is spatially structured. As George Lipsitz argues for the privilege based on inheritance of home ownership through the history of housing discrimination, "Opportunities in society are both spatialized and racialized" (Lipsitz 2007, 12). The racialization of space functions through the exclusion and exchange of value, and the value that determines the racial meaning of places affects the racialization process. This white spatial imagination is "a central mechanism for skewing opportunities and life chances in the United States along the racial lines" (Lipsitz 2007, 13).

Thus, through the historical lineage and the present state, the farmworkers and farmers become the context where racialized bodies enter space, and the space becomes racialized. The racialized bodies enter a space that has an extractive nature that reduces "life to a capitalist resource conversion" (Gómez-Barris 2017, xvi). Mexican labor and bodies function as the necessary subwhite agent for producing United States-American fruit and vegetable consumption. México, as a region, also becomes part of this white spatial imaginary, where these bodies of cheap labor are located and reduced for the functioning of racial capitalism. México is, therefore, the site of extraction; Mexicans are the primary labor extracted for the sake of producing a cheap competitive product, which dialectically affects the economies of other countries, namely México, continually dislodging Mexican farmworkers and Indigenous groups from their lands due to the United States's economic monopoly on the market.

Thus, the Mexican farmworker operates as a manifestation of racial extractivism, exploited for labor and yielding inexpensive agricultural goods while being denied fair treatment comparable to that of white men. These colonial narratives shed light on why such mistreatment persist, as they are influenced and sustained by ideologies rooted in white supremacy. Embedded within the backdrop of US imperialism's colonial past, the marginalization and neglect, particularly in terms of paths towards citizenship and permanent labor, underscore the sense of otherness associated with the in-between racial status of the Mexican body.

CONCLUSION

Hand harvesting still accounts for approximately 50 percent of fruits and vegetables in the United States. These fruits are carefully selected manually to determine the plant's readiness, given the emphasis on unblemished produce for maximizing profits. Yet, the farmworker remains expendable, as racial capitalism requires a surplus of workers, and the cheaper the labor, the more the profit, which entangles consumers in the farmworkers' precarity and their extraction of labor from their lands. As for consumers, some movements have advocated for fair trade food certification, such as Fair Trade Certified, which aims to combat poverty, advocate for workers' rights, promote gender equality, create resilient communities, and protect the environment.[9] At the same time, although these initiatives represent progress, their widespread adoption, accessibility, affordability, and emphasis on domestically grown produce rather than internationally sourced alternatives still are certainly not the norm. Hence, despite the rising popularity and demand for these products, the focal point remains affordability, a factor largely contingent on inexpensive labor. Yet, as one of the many plausible solutions, a demand for transparency between these food production sites and the consumer's political advocacy for more just systems remains viable.

9. "Fair Trade Certified—Sourcing Program from Fair Trade USA," Fair Trade Certified Website: https://www.fairtradecertified.org/.

While consumer accountability is a factor, the primary responsibility and culpability lies with those who uphold immigration regulations and national and international agricultural geopolitical trading methods, who often have little regard for the well-being of the most marginalized individuals. Consumer awareness and even small businesses' change toward more just practices will not alone change the global political and economic circumstances perpetuating these conditions, nor will it address the racial dynamics embedded in these systems. Thus, shifting our perspective of Latinxs and Indigenous farmworkers' dire circumstances to an analytic of racial extractivism allows us to begin untangling and unearthing the racial logics and white supremacist imaginaries that sustain and fortify this consumption of labor. In the United States, it is salient for food justice and environmental advocates to emphasize the discourse surrounding farmworkers, given that daily fruit and vegetable consumption relies on these individuals historically positioned at the liminal periphery. Thus, discussions about food justice in the United States can only occur by centralizing the farmworkers, as they are the primary means by which we eat.

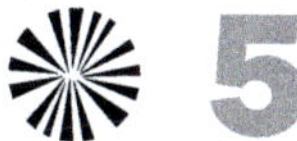 5

Intersectional Veganisms

Food, Gender, and Sexuality in the Veggie Mijas Collective

Jessica Ordaz

In July 2021, I conducted a preliminary research trip in Mexico City amid a global pandemic to start investigating the topic of this article. I ate at delicious vegan restaurants throughout the city and could not believe how many options there were. It had only been about ten years since I visited the city as a vegetarian—back then, the restaurant options were slim and the mock meat was mediocre. Enthusiastic to see the growth in options, I highlighted many of these businesses on my Instagram page. However, two kind strangers gave me a reality check. I had created a list of some of my favorite vegan restaurants thinking about the taste of the food and the ambiance of their locations. How naive. My post had over 730 likes and these two individuals were the only ones to mention that three out of the six businesses I highlighted were known for violating the rights of their employees. This included accusations of "wage theft, tip theft, overtime pay theft, worker abuse, and discrimination based on skin color and social class."[1] I was mortified. I should have thought about working conditions before amplifying these restaurants, which I knew nothing about other than that I enjoyed the taste of their food. I start with this anecdote because it highlights how veganism can and has become depoliticized, trendy, and mainstream, topics I will discuss throughout this chapter. This was a reminder that veganism is something to be practiced as much as theorized.

A BRIEF HISTORY OF VEGANISM

There are many reasons people go vegan: the environment and climate change, compassion for animals, protest of factory farming, an anticapitalist position, and for one's health and well-being. The oral histories I highlight throughout this article demonstrate that Black, Indigenous, and People of Color (BIPOC) knowledge about food, the environment, and animality, or "the social conditions of nonhuman animals," is central to understanding veganism today (Ko 2019, xvii). This chapter is influenced by the existing literature on veganism from authors of color. I am indebted to the work of A. Breeze Harper, Julia Feliz Bruek, Aph Ko, and Syl Ko. My use of interviews is intended to amplify vegan voices of color and decenter a mainstream vegan movement that is often viewed as white and middle class.

Although plant-based eating has been practiced throughout the world for ages, it was not until 1944 that Donald Watson and Elsie Shrigley, founders of the United Kingdom's Vegan Society, coined the term "vegan" (Dunham 2020, 43). They defined the concept as "a way of living that seeks to exclude, as far as possible and practical, all forms of exploitation of, and cruelty to, animals for food, clothing, and any other purpose" (Brueck 2017, 2). The term "veganism" might have started from a privileged, white-centered place, but as the following case studies demonstrate, communities of color have been engaging with questions of animal, human, and plant relations for centuries. The commodification of plants and other food sources was a key part of the European colonization of the

1. Veggie Mijas Post, Instagram, July 26, 2021.

Americas. The subsequent expansion of settler colonialism and empire-building transformed Indigenous foodways that included what we could consider vegetarian or vegan foods today. Veganism has been imagined and perhaps remembered and coded as white. Decentering whiteness and critically interrogating and historicizing intersectional veganism allows a new story to emerge. As food historian Jeffrey Pilcher argues, "food matters, not only as a proper subject of study in its own right, but as a captivating medium for conveying critical messages about capitalism, the environment, and social inequality to audiences beyond the ivy tower" (Pilcher 2012, xvii). In other words, food history reveals societal ideologies about identity, class, and culture.

SIGNIFICANCE

Out of the 332,403,650 people who live in the United States, approximately 9.7 million practice vegetarianism, including one million vegans.[2] According to a *Los Angeles Times* article published in 2020, veganism has become increasingly popular among a growing Latinx community. Patricia Escarcega argues that although "Mexican vegan cooking has its own cultural underpinnings . . . its recent popularity overlaps with the ascendence of veganism around the globe." She emphasizes that "the epicenter of the Mexican vegan explosion is Southern California, where in the last several years, weekly vegan food fairs in cities such as Los Angeles, Long Beach, Santa Ana and Ontario have been meeting a growing demand for plant-based Mexican vegan cooking."[3] While these cities are some of the most vegan-friendly in the United States, I argue that eating plant-based foods is not only ancestral (rather than a new trend), but that Southern California is only one of many places where Latinx veganism is practiced. To explore this and the various ways in which Latinx people are expanding the culture of veganism while drawing on traditional food practices, I conducted several interviews with Latinx vegans across the United States.

2. All Y'all's Foods, "Vegan Statistics 2022 (USA)," https://allyallsfoods.com/vegan-statistics-usa/.

3. Patricia Escarcega, "Mexi-Vegan Cooking is Mainstream in Southern California," *Los Angeles Times*, June 26, 2020.

The various threads in veganism, animal liberation, health, and the environment are all topics that have been of concern for Latinx folks for centuries. While issues such as climate change have recently invigorated more people to make critical and informed choices about what they consume, similar ideas and relationships with our surroundings have a much longer history throughout the Americas.

VEGGIE MIJAS AND INTERSECTIONAL VEGANISM

I co-founded the Denver Metro chapter of Veggie Mijxs during the height of the COVID-19 pandemic in 2020. After experiencing a very white and mainstream vegan movement in Denver, Colorado, and then lockdowns that made life further isolating and insular, I decided to help create intersectional spaces that would allow for the growth of a community, even if virtual for the moment. The Denver chapter was part of a national collective founded in 2018, Veggie Mijas. Veggie Mijas, a "women of color/trans folks of color/gender non-conforming collective for folks that are plant-based or are interested in a plant-based lifestyle that have marginalized identities and/or experiences with food insecurity/food apartheids," started as a recipe-sharing website.[4] Since then, it has grown into a collective with over ten chapters throughout the United States.

The collective was co-founded by Mariah Bermeo and Amy Quichiz with the aim of sharing plant-based resources for BIPOC and the LGBTQIA+ community. Quichiz, who has Colombian and Peruvian roots, writes that she "wanted to create a place where folks of color [could] speak about veganism without having to go through . . . turmoil like [she] did when . . . navigating these spaces."[5] The need to create a BIPOC-focused collective speaks to the inaccessibility of the larger mainstream white vegan movement. Of particular interest to organizers is the decolonization of food and an approach that is nonshaming and encouraging of BIPOC who have felt excluded from the mainstream vegan movement.

---

4. Veggie Mijas, https://www.veggiemijas.com/mission.

5. Angela Melero, "Veggie Mijas Founder Amy Quichiz Turned a Vegan Potluck into a Full-Blown Movement," July 25, 2022, https://www.thezoereport.com/wellness/veggie-mijas-founder-amy-quichiz.

The group's overall goal is to foster "a plant-based revolution using ancestral recipes—to feed themselves, their communities, and la cultura."[6] I had the privilege of speaking with several Veggie Mijas members and earth activists, as they call themselves, who spoke about their intersectional vegan activism. The following stories highlight the intersectional experiences of women and nonbinary folks in vegan culture and their relationships with food justice.

CASE STUDY #1: WHITE VEGANISM

Many people I interviewed discussed how difficult it is to center race and ethnicity when organizing around mainstream veganism. In 2020, Alejandra Tolley, a twenty-two-year-old Mexican American and vegan of three years, recounted her experiences growing up near Los Angeles. Tolley turned to vegetarianism after watching the documentary *Food Inc.* in high school and became vegan after learning more about the dairy industry. Tolley's early activism included attending protests against circuses, but the organizing strategies and tactics made her uncomfortable. "Violently screaming at attendees, including kids, was abusive," she said. Frustrated by the lack of conversations about what it meant to let go of cultural ties to food, Tolley joined Veggie Mija. Now an organizer with the collective, Tolley appreciates that members think differently about "connecting to the earth, animals, and the environment, through a black and brown intersectional lens." One of the projects organized by the local Los Angeles chapter is the establishment of community fridges in areas where food insecurity is high. This collective has been of particular significance to Tolley because she experienced the harm that single-issue approaches can cause.[7]

On August 10, 2019, Tolley attended the Los Angeles Animal Rights March. She wrote "dismantle white veganism" in red letters on a sign and proudly displayed it at the event. Her thinking was that "there need[ed] to be a radical shift in the (vegan) movement," one that connects the "systemic

---

6. Hannah Rose Mendez, "Reimagining Our Recipes, Preserving Our Histories," *Atmos*, December 13, 2022, https://atmos.earth/reimagining-recipes-preserving-histories-veggie-mijas-ancestral-foods/.

7. Alejandra Tolley, interview with author, Diamond Bar, California, November 2, 2020.

failures that produce lack of accessibility to healthy foods." She wanted to emphasize that food is political and that veganism should be connected to workers, environmental racism, and animals. When the marchers arrived in downtown Los Angeles, one of the event's staffers approached Tolley and asked her to put down the sign because it was discriminatory. She was then asked to leave the event. When she didn't, marchers started to come up to her angrily. Feeling unsafe, she decided it was time to leave. After leaving the event and going home, Tolley posted a photo of the protest sign, with some added text, on her Instagram page. The caption stated that a white man had told her not to get color involved in animal rights. She went to bed and the next morning awoke to hundreds of frightening comments on the Instagram post. Some people attacked her on a personal level and others claimed the post was racist. Tolley shared that this response is typical of the mainstream white vegan movement. "White people made themselves the victims and felt attacked instead of recognizing that white veganism is a system of whiteness," she said.[8] Utilizing an intersectional lens when theorizing and practicing veganism is essential in shifting the movement away from a single issue towards one that intersects across a multitude of issues and inequalities across the globe.

CASE STUDY #2: CLASS AND VEGANISM

Rebeca Cintron-Loaisiga, a Boricuan culture and history educator, lives in Camden, New Jersey, and had been practicing a plant-based lifestyle for over nine years at the time of our interview. A mother of two children, she became vegan while searching for healthy foods. Having grown up eating traditional Puerto Rican foods such as beans, rice, canned meats, and root veggies, Rebeca hoped to incorporate more plant-based foods for her family. Not being around vegan organizations when she first went vegan, she was excited to become the Philadelphia organizer for Veggie Mijas. In this capacity, she has attempted to create "space to exist and explore plant-based foods" while "not forc[ing] veganism on anyone, [or] preaching."[9]

---

8. Tolley interview.

9. Rebeca Cintron-Loaisiga, interview with author, Camden, New Jersey, November 23, 2020.

In speaking with Rebeca about veganism and class, she emphasized the lack of accessibility to certain foods. For instance, she shared that it has been difficult to find vegan foods and consequently has at times resorted to shopping at Whole Foods, which means having a much smaller budget to feed a growing family. She says, "Everyone should have access to food that grows on the ground, but they don't." Her experiences with white veganism further demonstrate the tense relationship between food and class. She states that she was "welcome" into white vegan spaces as a non-Black Latinx vegan, but folks did not understand why she couldn't always attend farmer's markets in the suburbs. "It's more expensive than going to SaveAlot," she said.[10]

In addition to class differences, Rebeca does not support the aggressiveness of some white mainstream vegans who "force veganism down people's throats" and don't consider various cultural differences. For instance, she adds that she does not frown upon people using animals in ceremonial practices. "The issue is killing animals in large quantities and for no reason," she continues. Mainstream veganism is so white that when Rebeca first went vegan, she thought a white man invented it! Yet, she says that she has learned that "plant-based foods are ancestral. Plant-based eating is from the earth."[11]

CASE STUDY #3: THE GEOGRAPHY OF FOOD SCARCITY

Chicana, queer, and the daughter of a single mother, Daniela Medrano was born and raised on both the Northside and Southside of Chicago. She is thirty-one years old and has a bachelor's degree in philosophy and sociology. She identifies as a feminist, socialist, and, according to her family, *una rebelde*. Having grown up in a working-class community and having spent a lot of her life visiting Mexico, Medrano was inspired to work with unaccompanied children and on immigration.[12]

Medrano stopped eating meat at the age of twelve after visiting a slaughterhouse with her father. She became vegetarian the moment she witnessed

---

10. Cintron-Loaisiga interview.

11. Cintron-Loaisiga interview.

12. Daniela Medrano, interview with author, Chicago, Illinois, November 27, 2020.

a cow being slaughtered in front of its calf. Then, as an undergraduate student at Oberlin College, she took an animal rights class. Her professor was a huge influence, as he turned her onto veganism. During this time, Medrano was also part of a vegan-friendly and people-of-color food co-op. She felt safe in this space and became increasingly passionate about animal liberation. However, the animal rights club she joined was very white. She participated for about one semester because she didn't connect with the organizers. Medrano shares that she "felt left out of the conversation [and that] the focus was more on animal cruelty than the impact that veganism had on people of color." At the co-op, she could "be [her] brown self before [she] was vegan," whereas in the vegan club, she felt judged. In retrospect, she admits that what she needed was for white vegans to understand that people of color have their own backgrounds and histories to consider before their veganism. She needed more nuance. For instance, Medrano now views her form of veganism as a form of resistance.[13]

Medrano was looking for intersectional veganism because that was her experience. She grew up eating a standard American diet because her mom worked three jobs. Meals included processed food, sausages, bologna, eggs, mac and cheese, and essentially anything she could prepare quickly and would feed four growing children. Her mom cooked beans, eggs, and tortillas. Similar to many working-class families, McDonald's was considered a treat. During special occasions, family gatherings consisted of meat-centered foods such as tamales, gorditas, and menudo. Once Medrano became vegetarian, she mainly ate nopales, avocados, and lentils.[14]

When Medrano transitioned to veganism, her mom initially thought it was a phase. She also became vocal about what people ate. "I was that vegan that wouldn't let you have a meal in peace without telling you the origins of it," she says. However, her approach shifted fairly quickly. Medrano is now a Chicago organizer for Veggie Mijas, where she hosts events on healing, self-care, and bike riding.[15]

---

13. Medrano interview.

14. Medrano interview.

15. Medrano interview.

Medrano is particularly interested in issues of food scarcity and insecurity because they intersect with racism. The layout and segregation of Chicago have impacted the access people have to food and grocery stores in particular—a key factor white vegans missed during her college experience, she asserts. She currently lives in a predominantly Latinx working-class family neighborhood on the Northside. Her family lives in the Southside and she points out the limits of public transportation, which does not extend all the way south, making it more challenging to access grocery stores with quality and fresh foods. The train system is centered downtown. Yet the number of grocery stores depends on what region one lives in. All the Trader Joe's stores are on the Northside. Living in a neighborhood with few grocery options means one must drive to avoid lower-quality foods. In poor regions, there are more liquor stores than grocery stores. "There is no investment in [working-class] communities," she says. Medrano points out that there are bridges and "invisible borders" that divide entire communities.[16]

CASE STUDY #4: VEGAN BRUJERIA

Monica Divane is also an organizer for Veggie Mijas. She started the Orlando chapter in 2019 and currently lives in central Florida. Divane identifies as vegan, bisexual, an Indigenous Latina, and a bruja. She became vegan in 2005 after she started studying to become a veterinarian in college and developed a stronger connection with animals. She remembers attempting to eat chicken and throwing up because she remembered the animal that she had dissected for class earlier in the day. This experience sparked her to change her major to environmental studies and become vegan. She has been vegan for the last fifteen years alongside her entire family, including her husband and two children.[17]

Puerto Rican and Honduran foods such as rice, beans, and tortillas were part of most meals growing up for Divane. Throughout the last few years, she has participated in protesting Ringling Brothers, supported farm sanctuaries, and become an organizer for the Florida chapter of Veggie

16. Medrano interview.

17. Monica Divane, interview with author, Lakeland, Florida, December 3, 2020.

Mijas. She asserts, "Finding Veggie Mijas for me . . . oh my god . . . I felt seen. I was like, "I am not the only Latina that's vegan!"[18]

Divane's veganism is deeply connected to her spirituality, feminism, and the environment. As a bruja and queer pagan, Divane is committed to healing, taking care of Mother Earth, and living with respect, all ideologies that shape her veganism. Divane first came out when she was attending college in New York while having access to a community of queer pagans and a host of events such as Pagan Pride. She points out that she views veganism as an anti-oppression movement and lifestyle, yet mainstream veganism isn't always so. "A lot of people don't see how it's all connected," she says. Divane attempts to live a life being cognizant of the interconnections between food justice, the environment, and spirituality as well as issues of race, class, gender, and sexuality.[19]

Divane shares that she always felt connected to something she did not yet have a name for. This came to be her identity as a queer bruja. "I finally had a name for what was inside of me, a name for what I felt was inside and what I was doing," she asserts. She had a sense for Brujeria because she has been focused on healing since she was a child. Growing up with a Mayan father from Honduras allowed her to grow up with Indigenous culture such as the importance of storytelling. These experiences impacted her practice with Brujeria. She states that she "could not see [herself] harming a living being [such as consuming animal products] and also healing at the same time," energy work that she felt needed to be in alignment as she prepared for ritual and meditation.[20] As a practitioner of Brujeria who is vegan, Divane collects items she might need such as feathers if she finds them outdoors, but she does not harm animals or other people to obtain them. For instance, blood is sacred among the Maya, but she only uses her own blood, collecting in moments such as when she gets her blood drawn. "Blood is your life source," she says. Veganism is as important as Divane's multiple identities, as someone interested in magic and wonder, paganism, queerness, and beliefs outside the binary, all while centering her Latinx and indigenous roots.

---

18. Divane interview.

19. Divane interview.

20. Monica Divane, Brujeria Veganx, Season 1, Episode 4, 12/10/21

XICANX VEGANISM AND MESTISX MEDIA

Suzy González is a Veggie Mijas member, artist, and zinester. Their work epitomizes intersectional veganism. They self-identify as Xicanx, queer, pansexual, a vegan of more than ten years, a detribalized Indigenous person with Spanish roots, an empath, and radical.[21] González uses expressive arts to think through various topics, including ancestral foods. Based in San Antonio, Texas, González asserts that their "dedication to decolonizing consumption and art creation is intertwined with remembering the lessons that the earth has to teach us."[22] This vision is explored in their writing, art, and ideologies.

González writes that it is "through Xicanx Veganism, that [she] find[s] interest in the decolonization of one's diet, or a desire to reclaim the pre-colonial plant-based nourishment of [her] ancestors through food and herbal medicine" (González 2021, 44). They center Indigenous foodways in the development of veganism. But this was not always the case. When they first arrived at veganism, they protested animal exploitation alongside white vegans at venues such as circuses. They quickly realized that audiences would respond in anger. Feeling disheartened, González is now more interested in having conversations with people about food and culture. They state, "We don't have to use the V word [and] say things that turn folks off. [We] don't [have to] hold up a sign telling them they are evil."[23]

Instead, starting from the premise that "humans [were] spun from white and yellow corn" or the Mayan creation story, González has several art collections that are designed with literal and symbolic Mesoamerican meanings.[24] The art piece "Nature Nurtures" is a mixture of layered, dyed, and painted corn husks. González shares that "the corn husks represent the skin of the figures, recalling Mesoamerican beliefs that our very beings

---

21. Suzy González, interview with author, February 28, 2023.

22. Suzy González, https://suzygonzalez.com/page/1-ABOUT.html.

23. González interview.

24. Not Real Art, "Suzy González Paints the People of the Corn," https://notrealart.com/suzy-gonzalez/.

are created from *maiz*."[25] González has termed this process Mestisx media, which entails using materials intentionally and critically thinking through and grappling with how colonization plays into art materials. They hope their work decolonizes or re-Indigenizes art and all aspects of life.[26] While this work might not seem overtly vegan, they create art that centers plants and the earth with the dream that this will contribute to nonhuman animal liberation. In fact, González has redefined veganism as "a practice and ethics of care for animals, humanity, and earth."[27]

Thinking about various struggles, González uses this same medium to make overtly political statements about immigration enforcement. The 2017 art piece "Bridges Not Walls" and the 2019 piece "Close the Camps" are made from the same corn husks. Both of these artworks center on a future without institutions that create harm and separation. Centering ancestral mediums to make these statements is intersectional veganism in action.

Their latest exhibit, "Plantcestors" (2023), further demonstrates how intersectional veganism is about so much more than eating mock meats. The exhibit includes fourteen portraits of the community in San Antonio, Texas. Each portrait is based on the idea of plant nourishment and sustenance. González used plant materials that were identified as holding a deep connection to each person painted. She writes, "I believe that the plants we are connected to in this life are meaningful to us because they were meaningful to our ancestors. As we connect with our relative that is the land, we remember, we appreciate, and we reciprocate the gifts that she gives us."[28] The portrait of Diana Lopez is made from the pecans found in her family's land, mesquite pods, pericon, oil paint, and resin on the panel. Lopez states,

---

25. Not Real Art.

26. MALCS Radio, Platica con Suzy Gonzalez, https://soundcloud.com/chicana-latina-studies.

27. González interview.

28. Do 210, Plantcestors, https://do210.com/events/2023/2/18/plantcestors-paintings-by-suzy-gonzalez-tickets.

> Arboles de Nueces was where I grew up, each house was nuzzled with trees to calm the heat during the summer. I remember spending hours picking nueces right as the seasons changed. We stored them in 5-gallon buckets and when we traveled to Mexico we would share with my family. It brings tears to my eyes to remember those days and not be able to be in that place anymore. The houses and trees where we grew up were bulldozed to become unaffordable housing. My parents brought buckets of pecans with them. My family has been storing them and growing them for a future where we can once again live under the arboles.[29]

By centering plants from start to finish, González has created art that exemplifies intersectional veganism. Rather than repeat the spectacle of organizations such as PETA, González centers on connection, survival, and growth. They assert that their love for plants is as strong as their love for animals and argue that they have moved from a place of "critiquing the world" to "creating a world they want to see." Articulating a form of xicanx futurism, they state, "We get it, the world sucks [but] what's the world that we want yall, we got to dream it, and as artists, if we are not dreaming it and imagining it, what are we doing? If it's not beautiful people surrounded by plants, I don't know what it is."[30]

CONCLUSIONS

The life experiences and organizing strategies Veggie Mijas members shared demonstrate that Latinx voices must be a part of larger conversations around food politics, the environment, and animal liberation. Instead of adding to existing debates between mainstream vegans who claim that veganism is strictly about protecting animals and people of color who claim that veganism is a white issue, they show that there is a long history of plant-based foodways in the Americas and reframe veganism through an intersectional and decolonial lens and approach.

---

29. soozgonzalez, Instagram, https://www.instagram.com/p/CpF-BNTOPZF/.

30. González interview.

The experiences Veggie Mijas members highlighted in my interviews with them suggest that veganism is not confined to practices of whiteness. For Veggie Mijas members, veganism is an avenue to strengthen their ties to ancestral foods and practices, decolonization, and in some cases deepening their spirituality. The praxis of the collective, as women, trans, and gender nonconforming folks of color is redefining veganism as intersectional and crucial to calling out the violence of the food industry, food insecurity, and erasure of BIPOC activists in the food justice movement, often missed in mainstream white vegan spaces.

SECTION II

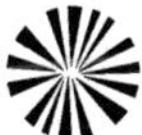

SOUTH AMERICA

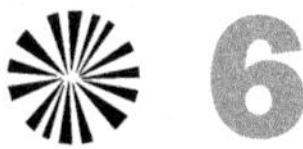 6

Marco Temporal
Deforestation in Service of Industrial Agriculture

Aline Silva, Bianca Mendes Rati, and Kigéw Puri

The 2022 Food and Agriculture Report of the United Nations forecasts that Brazil will soon become the largest cattle exporter, surpassing the United States (FAO 2022, 3). Livestock production generates profit for agribusiness at a very high cost for nonhumans and all Brazilians, especially the most marginalized populations and Indigenous peoples. The earth itself also pays the price. For instance, the Amazon rainforest has been desecrated by profitable industries such as logging, mining, cattle grazing, and ranching. This chapter will focus on the most destructive: deforestation in service of the agriculture industry and its devastating impact on the Amazon rainforest and on Indigenous foodways. One legal instrument used to facilitate the deforestation of the Amazon is the *marco temporal.* The article discusses how the *marco temporal* reflects colonialism's longstanding use of law to evict Indigenous people from their lands and how this concept, seemingly just a matter of property law, prioritizes food production for profit over food production by and for those who need it.

The first section enumerates the detrimental social, health, and economic effects of the deforestation of the Amazon. The second and final section analyzes how the concept of *marco temporal* has been weaponized in the courts to provide legal validation for agribusinesses' practices. This systemic exploitation not only uproots Indigenous communities but also perpetuates a cycle of environmental degradation in the Amazon, highlighting the deeply entrenched ties between profit-driven policies and the disenfranchisement of traditional food systems. The insidious intertwining of profit-driven motives with Indigenous land expropriation within the context of colonial practices unveils a harrowing narrative of displacement and ecological turmoil, showcasing the pernicious repercussions of privileging commercial harvests over communal sustenance.

The second-worst year on record for accumulated deforestation over the past fifteen years was 2022. The forest has lost the equivalent of nearly three thousand soccer fields per day.[1] Additionally, 2021 records show that 93 million cattle were in the region,[2] and cattle grazing is responsible for 75 percent of all Amazon deforestation.[3] Although deforestation itself is the most visible effect of the cattle industry, it has caused many other fatalities.

Industrial cattle ranchers and agribusinesses justify the costs of deforestation and the destruction of our forests by stating that Brazil "feeds the world." Meanwhile, 60 percent of the country's human population suffers from some type of food insecurity and apartheid.[4] Disturbingly, the industry is actively responsible for creating and maintaining hunger. While it is true that Brazil is a major exporter of agricultural products, including beef, soybeans, and other commodities, it is important to consider the

---

1. "Amazônia Perdeu Quase 3 Mil Campos de Futebol Por Dia de Floresta Em 2022, Maior Desmatamento Em 15 Anos," *Imazon*, January 18, 2023.

2. Aldem Bourscheit, "Crescimento Explosivo Da Boiada Na Amazônia Desafia Corte Nas Emissões de Metano Pelo Brasil," *InfoAmazonia*, November 9, 2021.

3. "Pastagem Ocupa 75% Da Área Desmatada Em Terras Públicas Na Amazônia," *IPAM Amazônia*, October 27, 2021.

4. "2º Inquérito Nacional sobre Insegurança Alimentar no Contexto da Pandemia da Covid-19 no Brasil," *Rede PENSSAN*, 2022: https://pesquisassan.net.br/2o-inquerito-nacional-sobre-inseguranca-alimentar-no-contexto-da-pandemia-da-covid-19-no-brasil/.

impacts of these activities on both the environment and the local population. It is important to recognize that the "feeding the world" argument used to justify deforestation often prioritizes profit over sustainability and equitable food distribution. Addressing food insecurity and apartheid in Brazil requires a holistic approach that considers the social, environmental, and economic impacts of industrial agricultural practices. Sustainable farming methods, land rights for indigenous communities, and policies that support small-scale agriculture can help address these issues while also promoting food sovereignty and environmental conservation. As international buyers like China, the United States, and the United Kingdom offer lucrative deals, Brazilian agribusinesses sell its products to them. This promotes food shortages and higher prices for Brazilians everywhere (Junior and Goldfarb 2021, 16).[5] These profitable deals are not only a threat to people of Brazil, but also its fauna. The second-largest meat-producing and exporting country in the world prioritizes selling to powerful and dangerous buyers from the global north.

Wildlife in the Amazon rainforest is increasingly under the threat of extinction. Today, more than ten thousand different species of Amazonian fauna are losing their natural habitats, access to food, or clean water due to illegal fires and deforestation led by the cattle industry and agribusiness.[6] The approximately 93 million cattle in the region, raised only to be murdered and be exported elsewhere,[7] amount to 9.3 times more than the number of specimens of any other one species—human or nonhuman. Their invasive farming produces pollutant gases, harming surrounding communities, the atmosphere, waterways and streams, and the fauna itself.

Of all populations impacted by the destruction caused by the cattle industry and agribusinesses, Indigenous peoples of the region endure the most harm. Currently, they are forcibly being pushed out of their territory

---

5. Victor Ohana, "Fila Da Fome Em Cuiabá Recebeu Ossos de 'Qualidade', Diz Governador de Mato Grosso," *CartaCapital*, August 1, 2022.

6. Stephen Eisenhammer and Oliver Griffin, "Mais de 10 Mil Espécies Correm Risco de Extinção Na Amazônia, Diz Relatório," *CNN Brasil*, July 14, 2019.

7. Débora Pinto, "Amazônia é Importante Para 81% Dos Eleitores, Revela Pesquisa," *((O))Eco*, September 5, 2022.

and face constant violence, expropriation, exploitation, and the threat of genocide. There are more than three hundred groups of Indigenous peoples living in the forest, totaling four hundred forty thousand residents.[8] The Yanomami people are the largest population in the forest. They are currently dealing with a humanitarian crisis of food scarcity and malnourishment, murders, and malaria due to the criminal actions of the mining industry.[9] The lands of the Uru-Eu-Wau-Wau, Jacareúba/Katawixi, Munduruku, and Araribóia peoples lost 215 acres just between July and August 2022.[10] Deforestation in Indigenous territory (TIs) in the Brazilian Amazon led to the emission of 96 million tons of carbon dioxide (CO2) between 2013 and 2021.[11] Violence against Indigenous peoples in Brazil increased in 2022, recording 416 cases of murder, 467 cases of violence against their territories, 158 cases of conflicts over land, and at least twenty recorded cases of sexual violence against children, adolescents, and Indigenous women.[12]

Brazilians living in cities, making up more than 84 percent of the population, are also affected by the climate changes and tragedies caused by the imbalances in the Amazon rainforest. As the forest controls all South American rain, moisture, and waterways, deaths caused by excessive rainfall, floods, and landslides in 2022 alone represented 25 percent of all deaths from these causes recorded between 2011 and 2022.[13] In addition,

---

8. "Os Povos da Floresta," *Instituto Sociedade, População E Natureza (ISPN)*, 21 July 2021.

9. "Na Amazônia, Um Povo Indígena Luta Pela Sobrevivência," *Nações Unidas Brasil*, August 10, 2022.

10. "Terras Indígenas Com Povos Isolados Na Amazônia Sofrem O Maior Ataque Do Ano," Instituto Socioambiental (ISA), September 26, 2022.

11. Ludmilla Souza, "Desmatamento Em Terras Indígenas Provocou Emissão de CO2 Na Amazônia," *Agência Brasil*, May 4, 2023.

12. Tiago Miotto, "Em 2022, Intensificação Da Violência Contra Povos Indígenas Refletiu Ciclo de Violações Sistemáticas E Ataques a Direitos," *Conselho Indigenista Missionário*, July 26, 2023.

13. Fernanda Luisa Martins Vasconcelos Filiú, Kathleen Gomes Vieira, and Liara Luiza Durigon Pozzobon, "Os Desastres Brasileiros E Suas Relações Com as Mudanças Climáticas," *Unicef Brasil*," October 4, 2022.

fires in the Amazon lead to fifteen million cases of respiratory and heart disease per year, and Indigenous territories absorb about a third of pollutants expelled by fires.[14] Air pollution especially impacts lower class and marginalized Brazilians, most of whom are descendants of historically and currently enslaved persons and the products of miscegenation[15] incited by the European church and its colonizers. Finally, climate, food, and Indigenous activists, prolabor politicians, and environmentalists are constantly in danger. Brazil is the country with the highest number of murders of environmentalists around the world over the past decade.[16]

These marginalized Brazilians living in rural and urban areas also suffer the consequences of the cattle industry and agribusinesses unethical and murderous practices. People who depend on rural work and small family farms often have their lands and settlements taken.[17] Cattle ranching and grazing, monocultural farming, and illegal land use desecrate real lives: the soil becomes unproductive and rural workers lose their means of livelihood. More often than not, rural workers do not have access to the food they produce and are food insecure themselves. In addition to social, food, and economic insecurity, rural workers are threatened with pesticide poisoning in the workplace. This represents half of the more than fourteen thousand cases confirmed by the Ministry of Health in the last decade, but this number only concerns reported

---

14. Ana Botallo, "Incêndios Na Amazônia Levam a 15 Milhões de Casos de Doenças Respiratórias E Cardíacas Por Ano." *Folha de S. Paulo*, April 6, 2023.

15. In Brazil, by the end of the eighteenth century, descendants of enslaved peoples were most of the population. Therefore, racist governments of the time installed a series of whitening policies by incentivizing lower income class European immigrants to come work in Brazil. These policies also glamorized racial mixing of the lower classes, creating the myth of a racially democratic country. See more at Sales Augusto dos Santos and Laurence Hallewell, "Historical Roots of the 'Whitening' of Brazil," *Latin American Perspectives* 29, no. 1 (2002): 61–82.

16. Fernanda Mena, "Brasil é País Mais Letal Da Década Para Defensores Da Terra E Do Ambiente, Diz ONG," *Folha de S. Paulo*, September 28, 2022; and press release, "Almost 2,000 Land and Environmental Defenders Killed between 2012 and 2022 for Protecting the Planet," *Global Witness*, September 13, 2022.

17. Mauricio Torres and Diana Aguiar, "A Boiada Está Passando: Desmatar Para Grilar," *Agro é Fogo*, January 16, 2023.

cases, as companies hide the real data and use no-regulated labor.[18] Workers from the cattle industry are at a higher risk for accidents, bone and muscular diseases,[19] as well as emotional distress due to poor working conditions (Cruvinel, Cruvinel, and Gomes 2022, 5). In the face of so much destruction and so many victims, one might ask why the cattle industry and agribusinesses are so prevalent in Brazil. One answer is that their economic power is guaranteed by historical political structures, capitalist labor practices, and neoliberal and white-supremacist ideology. Currently of the five hundred congressional members of the Brazilian chamber, three hundred are part of a political group influenced by the rural lobby.[20] Agribusiness giants in Brazil maintain a strong lobbying presence in Congress and have secured significant wins, such as passing legislation undermining Indigenous land rights and slashing regulations on pesticides.[21] The agribusiness lobby's think tank, IPA, employs strategies like spreading fake news and crafting talking points to advance its legislative agenda.[22] The IPA is intimately connected with the agribusiness caucus, sharing the same address and supported financially by agribusiness associations like the National Confederation of Agriculture, which in turn are backed by large multinational companies.[23] The IPA plays a pivotal role in creating

---

18. Bruno Fonseca, Pedro Grigori, and Thays Lavor, "Empresas Escondem Intoxicações de Trabalhadores Rurais Por Agrotóxico," *Repórter Brasil*, September 21, 2020.

19. Vanessa Ramos, "Ritmo Produtivo Extenuante Em Frigorífico Da JBS Causa Doenças Ocupacionais, Diz Justiça Do MS," *Brasil de Fato*, June 19, 2023.

20. Hugo Souza, "Bancada Ruralista Chega a 324 Deputados, Por Hugo Souza." Jornal GGN, August 30, 2023. https://jornalggn.com.br/congresso/bancada-ruralista-chega-a-324-deputados-por-hugo-souza/.

21. "Brazil's Supreme Court Rejects the Marco Temporal, but the Fight for Indigenous Land Rights Continues," Amazon Watch, October 13, 2023, https://amazonwatch.org/news/2023/0922-brazils-supreme-court-rejects-the-marco-temporal-but-the-fight-for-indigenous-land-rights-continues.

22. Larissa Mies Bombardi, and Audrey Changoe, "Toxic Trading: The EU Pesticide Lobby's Offensive in Brazil," Edited by Helen Burley, Seattle to Brussels Network, Friends of the Earth, 2022, https://friendsoftheearth.eu/wp-content/uploads/2022/04/Toxic-Trading-EN.pdf.

23. Cristiane Fontes, "What Will the Agribusiness Lobby Do Next?" *Sumaúma*, April 5, 2023. https://sumauma.com/en/como-a-alianca-entre-o-agronegocio-e-o-congresso-atua-para-garantir-o-retrocesso-na-legislacao-socioambiental-do-brasil/.

consensus and providing technical support to lawmakers, even drafting bills and paying journalists to influence public debate.[24] The agribusiness lobby, despite facing opposition from civil society and international pressure, has been able to advance its agenda through its significant influence and lobbying efforts. In other words, they are financed by the cattle industry and agribusinesses, and they compose 58 percent of the legislative voting power in Brazil. Today, agribusiness entities actively lobby against the demarcation of Indigenous lands and land reform, as well as against stricter labor regulation laws and anti-deforestation efforts in the Amazon and Pantanal (Pompeia, 2021, 283).[25] While agribusiness is lobbying and moving fast, in Indigenous demarcated territories, under fierce protection, deforestation has been decreasing by an average of 66 percent (Baragwanath and Bayi 2020, 20499). The whole Brazilian population is bombarded through various media with propaganda in favor of the cattle industry and agribusinesses. Latin American television network Rede Globo has a nonstop campaign with the jingle "Agro is tech, Agro is pop, Agro is everything." The ad campaign does a great job masking the industry's bloody hands by linking the industry with different aspects of Brazilians lives in an exclusively positive manner.

Although the term agribusiness is relatively new and the cattle industry is but seventy years old, the exploitation of Brazilian lands for wealthy Northern customers abroad has been actively working against its local populations since the arrival of Portuguese colonizers and the church in the 1500s. In this so-called "new [found] land," there were valuable natural resources, and above all, there was an enormous availability of fertile land for sugarcane

---

24. Fernanda Wenzel, "Meet the Think Tank Behind the Agribusiness' Legislative Wins in Brazil," Mongabay Environmental News, January 30, 2024, h24. Fernanda Wenzel, "Meet the Think Tank Behind the Agribusiness' Legislative Wins in Brazil," Mongabay Environmental News, January 30, 2024, https://news.mongabay.com/2024/01/meet-the-think-tank-behind-the-agribusiness-legislative-wins-in-brazil/.

25. The Pantanal is a complex of ecosystems that extends across Brazilian, Paraguayan and Colombian territories and that is recognized by UNESCO as a Natural Heritage of Humanity and Biosphere Reserve. In the region there is a meeting between five biomes: Cerrado, Chaco, Amazon, Atlantic Forest, and Bosque Seco Chiquitano. This is the largest wetland reserve on the planet, home to at least 4,700 species, including 3,500 species of plants, 650 of birds, 124 of mammals, 80 of reptiles, 60 of amphibians and 260 species of freshwater fish.

monoculture. To be clear, Portuguese colonizers, under the sanction of the church, first enslaved African peoples by kidnapping them and forcing them to work in Brazil for the sole purpose of expanding the cultivation of the sugarcane industry. This was the first model for agribusiness.

If appropriately funded and with the right policies in place, small family farms and practices could thrive. In fact, it is important to note that while the cattle industry and agribusinesses farm to export, small family farmers are key contributors to Brazil's food system, the economy, and local ecosystems. Therefore, if we desire to protect and support rural workers and small farms, stop mass deforestation, and restore Indigenous sovereignty, we should actively fight to dismantle the cattle industry and agribusinesses as well as the system sanctioning and financing their current expansion and success.

MARCO TEMPORAL AND THE ERASURE OF INDIGENOUS LAND

To take this argument further, we can look at the case of the *marco temporal*, or "historical cut-off point," a legal thesis that threatens the right of Indigenous land demarcation.[26] The thesis argues that because the last version of the Brazilian constitution is from 1988, only lands that were occupied by Indigenous peoples at that time are valid as Indigenous lands. The thesis is used in legislation open by the cattle industry and agribusinesses against Indigenous communities to take over their lands and territories.[27] *Marco temporal* is not new. In 2023, the Brazilian Supreme Court was ready to vote on the issue after years of deliberation.[28] If it were to become law, several processes for Indigenous land demarcations would

---

26. Wenzel, "Meet the Think Tank"; and Rafael Moro Martins, "How the Marco Temporal (Historic Cut-off Point) Affects Indigenous Land Demarcation," *Sumaúma*, June 6, 2023, https://sumauma.com/en/como-o-marco-temporal-afeta-as-terras-indigenas-em-10-perguntas/.

27. Global Witness, "The Brazilian Law Threatening Indigenous Land Rights" July 20, 2021, blog, https://www.globalwitness.org/en/blog/brazilian-law-threatening-indigenous-land-rights/.

28. United Nations Human Rights Office of the High Commissioner, "Brazil: Supreme Court Ruling in Favour of Ancestral Land Rights," September 26 2023, https://www.ohchr.org/en/press-briefing-notes/2023/09/brazil-supreme-court-ruling-favour-ancestral-land-rights.

lose strength and the communities would be expelled from their territories. That would determine the future of Brazil's Indigenous peoples and, by extension, the world's forests, biodiversity, and our ability to mitigate the climate crisis. This attempt of erasure would only perpetuate centuries of forced displacement of Indigenous peoples during Brazil's long history of colonization and dictatorship.

The major lobbyists behind the *marco temporal* thesis are agribusiness owners, especially the ones involved in soy monoculture, exported as grain, oil, or animal food. This represented 103 million tons of soy in 2022.[29] Agribusinesses want to expand soy production even more to increase profits from this.[30] A remarkable example of the *marco temporal* effect is happening in the state of Pará. Soy farmers there are trying to prevent the demarcation of the Munduruku people's territory, Planalto Santareno. The Munduruku have had claim to this land since 2008, but the legal identification process has been dragging on since 2018.[31] In this case, the soy lobby is actively advocating for the implementation of the *marco temporal* in order to prevent the new recognition of Indigenous territories, with a particular focus on regions such as Pará.[32]

The economic pressure exerted by the soy and cattle industries is significantly impeding the demarcation of Indigenous lands, thereby directly impacting Indigenous communities who are fighting for their ancestral territories. The aggressive lobbying tactics employed by the agribusiness

---

29. "Subprodutos Da Soja: Conheça Os Destinos E Usos Da Soja," *Agroadvance*, March 24, 2023.

30. Rosana Cavalcante De Oliveira and Rogério Diogne de Souza E Silva, "Increase of Agribusiness in the Brazilian Amazon: Development or Inequality?" *Earth* (Basel) 2, no. 4 (December 14, 2021): 1077–1100, https://doi.org/10.3390/earth2040064.

31. "Terras Indigenas Com Povos Isolados Na Amazônia Sofrem O Maior Ataque Do Ano," Instituto Socioambiental (ISA), September 26, 2022, https://www.socioambiental.org/noticias-socioambientais/terras-indigenas-com-povos-isolados-na-amazonia-sofrem-o-maior-ataque-do.

32. Diego Junqueira e Hyury Potter, "Marco temporal: apetite da soja por terras indígenas ignora pressão global contra desmatamento" *Brasil de Fato*, June 21, 2023, https://www.brasildefato.com.br/2023/06/21/marco-temporal-apetite-da-soja-por-terras-indigenas-ignora-pressao-global-por-desmatamento.

sector, including associations representing soy producers, are aimed at influencing key decision-makers in the congress, government, and judiciary, as well as attempting to sway the upcoming Supreme Court ruling on the *marco temporal*. The struggle for Indigenous lands is facing staunch resistance from soy producers across various regions of Brazil, raising serious concerns about the preservation of the environment and the protection of Indigenous rights. It is crucial to recognize that the outcome of the Supreme Court's decision on the *marco temporal* will have far-reaching implications for determining the traditional occupation of land by Indigenous communities and curbing the encroachment of soy producers on ancestral territories. In light of these developments, urgent action is needed to safeguard the rights and territories of Indigenous peoples against the undue influence of the soy lobby. It is imperative that we stand in solidarity with Indigenous communities and support their rightful claims to land and resources.

On September 21, 2023, the Supreme Court rejected the *marco temporal* thesis, but the Brazilian Senate decided to defy the Court and approve the law proposal anyway.[33] President Lula da Silva ultimately vetoed twenty of the law's twenty-two clauses. The two remaining mandate the following: the rights of Indigenous people do not override the interest of national defense and sovereignty policy; and the exercise of economic activities on Indigenous lands is permitted, as long as it is carried out by the Indigenous community itself—cooperation and hiring of non-Indigenous third parties is permitted so long as they are hired by Indigenous communities. Indigenous leaders say that the two clauses may intensify the harassment of Indigenous communities and undermine their sovereignty.[34] Still, the president's decision and support of the Supreme Court opens a path for the Indigenous movement to appeal if the situation changes for the worse. The lobbyists and pro-agribusiness groups will continue to try to pass this law. The *marco temporal* case illustrates very well the agribusiness articulation

---

33. "Brazil's Supreme Court Rejects the Marco Temporal."

34. Murilo Pajolla and Gabriela Moncau, "Marco Temporal: Veto de Lula Barrou Principais Retrocessos, Mas Pontos Sancionados Preocupam Indígenas E Indigenistas," *Brasil de Fato*, October 25, 2023.

of its political and economic powers to maximize profit over the life of all Brazilian life. It is a piece of legal artillery designed to destroy Indigenous lives and exploit the environment. As we will demonstrate even further, the setback of Indigenous peoples' rights is the first step towards environmental destruction. This exploitation of legal loopholes and political maneuvering opens the door to unfathomable consequences, not only for Indigenous communities but for the fragile balance of nature itself.

In this scenario, what does the recent election of deputies Célia Xakriabá and Juliana Cardoso Terena, the rise of former deputy Joênia Wapichana to the presidency of FUNAI, and above all, the creation of the Ministry of Indigenous Peoples under the leadership of elected federal deputy Sônia Guajajara mean for Brazilians? It is not surprising that, within less than six months of its existence, this ministry has already been subject to a maneuver to remove the authority over Indigenous land demarcation from its hands. And although the government has barely made progress in the demarcation of lands delayed by the Bolsonaro administration, it is already suspending the demarcation of new lands.[35] All of this is done under the shadow of the *marco temporal*.

These are clear examples of the liberal multiculturalism that Cusicanqui criticizes: for the first time in Brazilian history, Indigenous people are in the government's upper echelons, wearing their *cocares* and *graphisms*, but the material reality of Indigenous peoples and the threats to their rights remain as alive and dangerous as ever. One must wonder if the media conglomerates' depiction of Indigenous peoples as passive, spiritual helpers aiding in the emotional and economic growth of non-Indigenous people is yet another tactic of white supremacy acting behind the cattle and agribusiness industries today. One must wonder if this is not another attempt at subverting Indigenous sovereignty and derailing their struggle. The intricate web of oppression woven by white supremacy extends its threads even into the fabric of the cattle and agribusiness industries, as if seeking to silently strangle the roots of Indigenous autonomy and resilience, perpetuating a

35. Ana Carolina Amaral, João Gabriel, and Thiago Resende, "Governo Suspende Anúncio de Demarcação de Terras Indígenas Na Cúpula Da Amazônia," *Folha de S.Paulo*, August 8, 2023.

cycle of resistance against the forces that seek to exploit and erase their identity. It is a complex dance of power dynamics disguised within the operations of the cattle and agribusiness sectors, echoing a subtle yet potent echo of historical adversity and ongoing challenges faced by Indigenous communities that go to the heart of their fight for sovereignty and survival.

CONCLUSION

Preserving Indigenous culture, lifestyle, and sovereignty should be a communal goal for peoples across the globe, especially those settled in the Global North—if for nothing else, for the very selfish reason of wanting oneself and our loved ones to live in a flourishing world with abundant natural resources for all. It is clear now that Indigenous territories, although small, are responsible for holding back deforestation and the destruction of biodiversity, especially in the Amazon rainforest. When Indigenous people claim their right to land sovereignty, they are claiming an internationally recognized right to live in ancestral lands, in ways sustainable for themselves, their communities, and their natural environment. Never in their history have Indigenous Brazilians sought to engage in mass destruction of the earth or the fauna. Their deep-rooted reverence for nature and their ancestral connections imbue them with a profound sense of stewardship, driving a legacy of conservation that stands as a testament to their harmonious coexistence with the land. Most importantly, by opposing the cattle ranching and agribusiness industries, Indigenous peoples of Brazil are claiming their given right to protect what is still alive in the world and to heal what has been desecrated by the insatiable greed of a small group of people. In that way, they preserve the possibility of life itself (Krenak 2019, 49).

The demarcation of Indigenous lands is the shield of the forest. Studies and historical observation demonstrate that 90 percent of the conserved area of the Amazon forest corresponds to Indigenous lands and conservation units, which use sustainable methods for the maintenance of natural vegetation.[36] Such data prove that these territories play a decisive role in curbing deforestation and climate change. According to the Satellite

---

36. Cecilia Mayrink and Juliana Mello, "Terras Indígenas Funcionam Como Escudo Contra Desmatamento," *Agemt Jornalismo*, November 11, 2021.

Monitoring Project for Deforestation in the Legal Amazon (PRODES), between 2004 and 2014, there was an 80 percent reduction in deforestation in the area, mainly due to the creation of protected areas and control. The successful implementation of these conservation strategies highlights the effectiveness of combining Indigenous knowledge with modern technology to safeguard the Amazon's ecological balance and combat environmental degradation.

Brazilians cannot continue to rely on agribusinesses, the cattle industry, greedy corporations, or the three hundred congresspersons funded by their unethical dealings to feed Brazilians, take care of land where they operate, or work to preserve the Amazon rainforest. Rather, farming and agriculture should be viewed through an Indigenous lens. We should support local ethical producers on demarcated lands where food and land are sovereign and support their peoples. This would contribute to repairing the Brazilian food system, ensuring that foods are not used as weapons but rather equitably distributed to those on the margins and away from the most powerful. This approach is founded on principles of sustainability, respect for traditional knowledge, and creating a system where economic power is shared, envisioning a symbiotic relationship between the land, its resources, and the communities that depend on them.

The *marco temporal* concept has been used by agribusiness in Brazil to provide legal justification for their practices of land ownership and use. This concept suggests that Indigenous land rights are only applicable to territories that were occupied by Indigenous communities as of a specific date, which is often determined by the government. By using the *marco temporal* concept, agribusinesses can claim that Indigenous territories that were not occupied by a specific date are not entitled to legal protection, allowing them to expand their operations into these areas without facing legal challenges related to Indigenous land rights. The Brazilian government has been willing to go along with this concept in some cases, which has led to conflicts between Indigenous communities and agribusiness interests. Critics argue that this approach undermines Indigenous rights and contributes to environmental degradation.

The application of the *marco temporal* concept remains a complex and contentious issue in Brazil, with ongoing debates about its implications for Indigenous rights, environmental protection, and sustainable development. Our analysis, however, has sought to demonstrate that *marco temporal* is another chapter in a long legacy of colonialism in Brazil. The use of *marco temporal* effectuates through legal means the perpetuation of colonialist land theft, and it has environmental implications that are both local and global. It stands in the way of what we have suggested would be a more just, equitable transformation in Brazil's economy: namely, promoting a shift towards demarcating land as Indigenous, which would take it away from agribusiness and allow the flourishing of Indigenous food production practices that have, among other things, demonstrably been shown to reduce the devastating rates of deforestation that are destroying the Amazon.

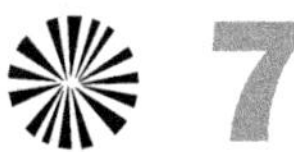

7

Guyanese Food's Global Entanglements

Dennis Saavedra Carquin-Hamichand

THROUGHOUT ITS HISTORY, Guyana has been marked by relentless movement and transformation. Its people, culture, and natural resources are in a constant state of flux, shaped by numerous internal and external influences (Ali 2020, 203–204). The catalysts behind this perpetual transformation include ongoing migrations and the impact of external influences such as colonization and neoliberalism. As Guyana endeavors to forge its identity, this state of flux persists, with Guyanese individuals engaged in an enduring "struggle for freedom," in the words of Vincent Harding in *There Is a River*.[1] Today, characterizing Guyana as engaged in a "struggle for freedom" could be contentious, given its projected status to be one of the most prosperous nations in the Caribbean and South America in the coming years (Ali and Schena 2017, 23–24; LaBennett 2024, viii, 2;

1. Vincent Harding's historical account emphasized that the initial phases of the Black struggle for freedom were characterized by a resolute resistance against European oppressors and their African allies. Their objectives were to safeguard their cultural traditions and cohesive societies, thwart the threat of fragmentation, and vigorously assert their autonomy and distinct identity while rejecting European hegemony and striving for a

Idrovo and Yanoff 2022). However, the persistent presence of influential external forces seeking to wield authority over vital institutions and corporations remains a formidable obstacle to achieving complete sovereignty. Guyana's considerable wealth, coupled with its inadequate infrastructure, has already attracted the influence of North American and Asian corporate interests in the nation.[2]

Like many cultures, Guyanese identity cannot be pinned down to one characteristic. Living in the interstices of multiple realities—South American, Asian, and African—Guyanese people's identity and existence are hybridized.[3] Living in these liminal spaces of Guyana, Asia, and Africa, Guyanese people are not defined by one dominating identity. We are not only Indian or African or Amerindian or Douglas or Christian or Hindu or Muslim. We are all these parts. And the composition of Guyanese identity continues to change today as more and more Venezuelans migrate to Guyana.[4] Even in the second diaspora outside of Guyana, the signifier Guyanese remains (Ali 2020, 204). The fluidity of our identity shifts and changes constantly and goes beyond the boundaries of one single reality. Our *creoleness* comes out of the hybrid/interstitial space we live in as a people and a nation. This hybrid reality unifies us.

---

future in line with their forebears' aspirations. Building upon Harding, this struggle's resonance can be discerned in the journey of Guyana, which endured centuries of colonization, and where the enduring spirit of this struggle remains palpable in the efforts to secure emancipation in August 1834 and, later, independence in May 1966 (Harding, 1981, 3–23).

2. Exxon, a major American company, *discovered* the Liza 1 oil field in Guyana in 2015, leading to significant investments of around $5 billion in oil production by 2020 (Padula et al. 2023, 13).

3. For more on hybridity, read Homi Bhabha's *The Location of Culture*, 1994; Antony Easthope, 1998, "Bhabha, hybridity and identity."

4. According to CARICOM, Guyana Secretariat Laurette Bristol, "In the first quarter of 2020, over 113,000 Venezuelans sought the safety of the Caribbean. Many of these persons are children and youth, representing 12% of the registered refugee population in Trinidad and Tobago and 31% of the refugee population in Guyana" (Bristol 2023, v). Since we share an open border with the neighboring countries when they are going through economic challenges, they move to Guyana, and now that Guyana is experiencing significant growth in its economy, more migrants are moving there to live, which is leading to a (re)shaping of the Guyanese identity.

Paradoxically, though, as these diverse influences unify to constitute "Guyanese identity," they remain distinct sociopolitical markers. For example, Guyana's current government has called its agenda "One Guyana." However, identity plays a role during political elections, allegiances are questioned, and racialized tensions are stoked. In this contradiction of unity and disunity, the Guyanese identity is formed. We know it is there even when we do not want to address it directly. Similarly, our food carries these sociopolitical markers of unity and difference (Rose 2023, n.p.; LaBennett 2024, 4–5).

In this chapter, I explore colonization's profound impact on Guyana's cultural landscape, tracing the transformation of Amerindian, African, Indian, and Chinese culinary traditions in the face of European exploitation. I delve into the resilience and adaptation of these communities, manifested through culinary innovations like Pepper Pot, Fufu, Metemgee, and Indo-Guyanese curry, which not only reflect the fusion of diverse influences but also serve as acts of cultural resistance and preservation amidst the enduring legacy of colonialism and neocolonial dynamics. In order to explore these focal areas, my approach will adopt a multidisciplinary methodology encompassing history, politics, philosophy, and culinary culture. This methodology aims to comprehensively examine the evolution of Guyanese cuisine, with a particular emphasis on understanding how it has been molded and continues to be influenced by colonial, postcolonial, and neocolonial forces.

When European colonizers began to construct their colonies on this land in the sixteenth century, what is today known as Guyana began to form. The arrival of colonialism initiated the change in culture, landscape, language, and ethnic identities (Ishmael 2013, 39–65). These colonizers did not plan this formation, since they primarily aimed to extract and exploit all they could from this land to develop Europe. Development, however, is suspect. As Walter Rodney, a Guyanese historian, stresses in his seminal work *How Europe Underdeveloped Africa*, before Europe engaged in their colonizing mission in the fifteenth century, Africa was being developed because development and utilization of natural resources from one's surrounding is natural to human existence as a means of survival (2011, 23). He writes that at the same time that Europe was developing,

European colonists were underdeveloping Africa by exploiting people and extracting resources to take back to Europe (28–29).[5] This same argument can be applied to the Guyanese context and all the colonies exploited by European colonizers. The agenda of the Dutch and British colonizers was to extract resources from this land to develop Europe—which is why they maintained the plantocracy for centuries. Their development also required enslaved and exploited laborers from Africa and Asia (Ishmael 2013, 92–102, 172–77).

Guyana's culture exhibits a constant state of transformation. Its small area (214,970 square kilometers) and population (814,000 people as of 2023) amplify the perceptibility of this ongoing evolution when contrasted with larger nations. The departure of individuals results in a palpable void within the community, while the arrival of newcomers equally engenders a noticeable presence. Historical records about the arrival of European colonizers emphasize the immediacy of this phenomenon, with documented sources underscoring the rapidity of this cultural movement (Richards-Greaves 2013, 77). In precolonial Guyana, the coastal regions were inhabited by various Amerindian tribes, including the Caribs, Akawois, Arawaks, Warraus, Macushis and Wapisianas, Arecunas, Patamonas, and the Wai-Wais (Ishmael 2013, 24–28), who had well-established communities for more than eleven thousand years (Edwards and Gibson 1979, 161–63; Ishmael 2013, 17). However, Dutch and British colonizers' exploitative and extractive agendas compelled the Amerindians to abandon their fertile ancestral homelands. They were forced to seek refuge in more remote and less hospitable hinterland areas within the Guyanese territory. In these newly adopted regions, the Amerindians transitioned into a nomadic way of life and were forced to innovate and devise new survival strategies (Schacht 2013, 15–16).

Donald Sinclair and Carolann Marcus showed that over centuries of living in relative isolation from coastal populations, Amerindian communities

---

5. Rodney explains that the imperialist system is primarily responsible for African underdevelopment, draining wealth and hindering rapid resource development. The system is manipulated by Western European capitalists, who have expanded their exploitation to Africa. Recently, US capitalists have joined and replaced them, benefiting workers in metropolitan countries who have benefited from the underdevelopment of Africa.

developed a profound symbiosis with the land. This relationship not only sustained their livelihood but also enriched their belief systems and preserved cultural traditions. Every aspect of Amerindian life, from their modes of dress to religious rituals, hunting practices, and culinary traditions, is intertwined with nature. Their profound understanding of the terrestrial world allowed them to master culinary and medicinal applications, reflecting a holistic approach to their environment. As a result, foods and culinary preparations emerged as inseparable from the identity and evolution of Amerindian communities (Sinclair and Marcus 2015, 76–85).

When the Europeans started colonizing Guyana, the Amerindians' dietary patterns underwent a significant transformation. In contrast to their prior reliance on fishing and fertile soil for planting in the coastal regions, the Amerindians were compelled to shift towards hunting and adapt their agricultural practices to suit the harsh conditions of the hinterland areas. This transition gave rise to notable culinary innovations, one of which is the pepper pot, currently esteemed as Guyana's national dish. This distinctive culinary creation is a savory meat stew characterized by its generous use of peppers and cassareep, an extract derived from bitter cassava, which is known for its preservative properties[6] (Schacht 2013, 15–29; DuFord 2012, 27–30). Notably, pepper pot's remarkable ability to be preserved for long periods without refrigeration has been attested by many Guyanese, with the consensus that it achieves an even more delectable flavor profile as it matures in the pot (Nelson 2010, 60–62). This movement and culinary development were one of Guyana's earliest developments in present-day cuisine (Richards-Greaves 2013, 84).

Pepper pot, for the Amerindians, is a sign of resilience and their will to survive. Throughout history, we have seen the genocidal actions of colonizers towards Indigenous people across the world. Living in a culture of genocide and exploitation imposed on them by the European colonizers, the Amerindians, like many other colonized peoples, found ways to

6. This popular ingredient possesses lethal properties. Consuming even small quantities of raw bitter cassava can be fatal. However, boiling nullifies its toxicity, transforming it into cassareep, a black-bittersweet syrup used widely as a flavoring sauce in Guyana (DuFord 2012: 27–30).

survive (Colwell-Chanthaphonh 2005, 114; Newton 2014, 6–7). This is why Indigenous communities often remind visitors to tell people that "We are still here" (Dai et al. 2023, 749–751). I heard this refrain when I visited some Mayan communities in Guatemala with a group of colleagues, and a similar process of recognizing the contributions of the Amerindians is taking place so that we can remember that they are still here.

As described before, the pepper pot symbolizes the vibrancy of the Amerindians in Guyana, reminding us that they are still here (Sanders 1995). Over time, it became part of Guyana's cultural identity. The need to find ways to survive led to many innovations for the Amerindians in their cuisine. Many stem from the use of cassava or yuca.[7] The versatility of cassava has become associated with the Amerindian identity and culture in Guyana.

Before rice and corn became common sources of calories, cassava was a staple food widely grown and eaten in Guyana. Even with the arrival of enslaved people, indentured laborers, and people from various ethnic backgrounds to work on plantations, cassava remained the primary food source

---

7. Cassava is categorized in two ways: sweet and bitter. Sweet cassava is used in many forms to make different foods that do not require any extraneous preparation procedures, for example, cassava pone (a sweet cake), sweet and savory cassava balls (boiled, mashed, rolled into balls, and fried), meat and egg balls (stuffed mashed cassava with meat or a boiled egg), "boil and fry," (this is eaten with salt fish or stews) farine (a cereal that can be eaten uncooked or made into porridge), and chips, among many other products. Many of these products are made from ready-to-eat sweet cassava, which requires boiling or frying. One would find sweet cassava or yuca in supermarkets in the United States (Thomas 2014). On the other hand, bitter cassava, not sold in US supermarkets, is commonly used in Guyanese cooking and produces various prized products. Cassareep and cassava flour or farine are the standouts since they are both integral components of pepper pot. Cassava bread is made from the leftover grated pulp after extracting the juice from the cassava using a matapee, a long cylindrical nibbi extractor. The leftover pulp is dried for a day or two, sifted, and then baked on a very hot grid. It can be enjoyed soft and hot, as favored by Indigenous communities, or it can be sun-dried for a few hours before being packaged and stored. The toxic juice extracted from the bitter cassava is boiled for several hours in a large pot. Throughout this process of homogenization, the top layer of "scum" or "skin" is constantly skimmed off as it comes to the surface until that being boiled is thick, tacky, and of a pure dark brown, almost black look and becomes the pure, unadulterated cassareep—one of the finest and most sought-after condiments in Guyanese cuisine (Balston 2020; Ewbank n.d.).

(Thomas 2014). It was crucial in connecting different ethnic communities nationwide, serving as a unifying staple food. The legacy of this food is seared into our consciousness; even as we eat pepper pot at Christmas time, we are reminded of its origins from the Amerindians, and it is something we cannot forget. As we claim it as Guyanese, we know it was birthed in the will to survive in the Amerindian context in Guyana, and it becomes a way for us to honor their legacy and contribution to the Guyanese cultural landscape. Despite the mainstream adoption of dishes like pepper pot, their roots in Amerindian culture remain known and celebrated. This cultural resilience is particularly significant in the face of encroaching fast-food chains, which threaten to overshadow traditional culinary practices.[8] In this context, food becomes a form of cultural resistance, a means of asserting and preserving identity amidst the tide of globalization and neoliberalism.[9]

A major contributor to Guyanese cuisine was the introduction of enslaved Africans brought to Guyana by the Dutch and British to work

8. In recent years, Guyana has experienced a noticeable influx of North American and Chinese corporations into its local market and established businesses—fast foods and supermarkets with imported processed foods. This phenomenon resembles what George Ritzer and Elizabeth L. Malone called "McDonaldization": "the process through which the principles of highly successful fast-food restaurants extend their dominance over various sectors of American society and an increasing number of societies worldwide. These principles revolve around efficiency, calculability, predictability, and control" (2000, 99).

9. Roland Robertson and Kathleen E. White see no universally accepted definition for globalization due to its recent emergence in academic and political discourse, with varying perspectives worldwide, especially in developing countries and across diverse cultural contexts. Some scholars even refer to "globalization" in the plural, recognizing its interdisciplinary nature and multiple processes (Robertson and White, 2006). Within this framework, neoliberalism arises as figures like Tejaswini Ganti advocate for economic reform policies, a market-centric development model, and an ideology valuing market exchange and competition. Neoliberal policies aim to deregulate the economy, liberalize trade and industry, and privatize state-owned enterprises. Neoliberalism carries significant economic, social, and political implications, influencing human action and replacing previous ethical beliefs (Ganti 2014, 90–91). The entry of fast-food giants such as KFC, Pizza Hut, Burger King, Starbucks, and Popeyes into Guyana's economy (surprising that McDonald's has yet to arrive) coincides with the nation's burgeoning oil industry under ExxonMobil's influence.

on the rice and sugar plantations.[10] We cannot discuss food development in Guyana without addressing the searing impact of the transatlantic slave trade on African communities and their cultural heritage, underscoring the inhumanity and the enduring trauma it caused (Harding 1981). The systematic violence endured by African populations in Guyana and the numerous British colonies throughout the transatlantic slave trade was predicated upon the dehumanization of enslaved Africans and the deliberate eradication of their cultural identities. Notwithstanding the concerted efforts of their oppressors, the resilience of the human spirit in safeguarding and perpetuating cultural, religious, and gastronomic facets of their heritage became patently evident. Enslaved Africans managed to preserve vestiges of their cultural, religious, and culinary traditions (Ortiz 1947, 97–110). Fernando Ortiz's description of Africans in Cuba exemplifies similar realities of enslaved Africans in Guyana. In summary, he states that the enslaved Africans arrived in Cuba without their culture, institutions, and tools, causing profound disconnection from their homelands. Unlike Indigenous people, who had hope of dying on their land, Africans were forcibly uprooted from their homes and subjected to hardships without the hope of a return. They lived in constant fear and longing for freedom, with thousands of Africans brought to Cuba over centuries. In contrasting the experiences of the whites and Blacks, Albert Memmi writes that both whites and Africans experienced varying degrees of disconnection, living together in an atmosphere of terror and oppression. This environment tore Black people apart, leaving them longing for justice and dignity (Memmi, Judaken, and Lejman 2021, 67–68; Ortiz 1947, 102–103).

In the contemporary context, the Afro-Guyanese culinary culture's movement towards freedom and justice is presented as a form of resistance. Preserving dishes like Fufu and Metemgee symbolizes the profound historical continuity between the precolonial, colonial, and postcolonial eras (Richards-Greaves 2013, 82–84). Michelle and Suzanne Rousseau, in

10. *New York Times* columnist Brent Staples described the sugarcane plantation industry as the "slaughterhouse of the trans-Atlantic slave trade by killing more people more rapidly than any other kind of agriculture." Staples, citing the Trans-Atlantic Slave Trade Database, "estimates that at least 70 percent of the 12 million or so captives who left Africa for the Americas on slave ships were destined for sugar colonies" (Staples 2018; Eltis 2018).

Provisions: The Roots of Caribbean Cooking, reiterate the often-ignored impact of African women[11] in preserving African cuisine, showcasing how "subsisting on food from provision grounds[12] demanded ingenuity, innovation, creativity, and practicality, particularly in the kitchen" (Rousseau and Rousseau 2018, 18). This creativity can be seen in Fufu and Metemgee, as culinary exemplars representing the strength and adaptability of African heritage in Guyana and the Caribbean. They highlight the ability to embrace the movement and changes in circumstances, taking on new features by incorporating new ingredients into their creation that match the present landscape. Fufu, crafted from a blend of starchy staples like cassava, yam, or plantains, has been a staple in diverse West African cuisines for generations (Houston 2005, 64). It is now part of Guyanese culture and identity. Similarly, Metemgee, a rich and complex one-pot meal, can be traced back to African culinary traditions and is now an integral part of Guyanese culinary culture (17, 111). Beyond their functional role as sustenance, these dishes embody a profound commitment to cultural preservation and the unwavering connection to the African cultural roots of the enslaved. Over time, these foodways underwent a process of syncretism, intermingling with various cultural influences, thereby forging distinctive culinary traditions that exemplify the adaptability and resilience of the African diaspora in the face of relentless adversity. Highlighting these two foods from the Afro-Guyanese community is part of the culture of *faithful witnessing*.[13] It is a way of preserving as much of the ancestral memory necessary to resist the culture of colonization.

---

11. Michelle and Suzanne Rousseau write that the culinary history of the West Indies can be traced back to the women who farmed, harvested, bartered, sold, prepared, manipulated, and redefined the ingredients available to them. The culinary history and life stories of Afro-Caribbean women are intertwined, beginning under the harsh conditions of a sugar plantation. These women developed culinary techniques and eating habits, which form the basis of the West Indian diet (Rousseau and Rousseau 2018, 18).

12. "Ground provisions" or "provision grounds" include roots, tubers, and starchy fruits, for example, cassava, yams, eddo, etc., from the small farms of the enslaved Africans (Rousseau and Rousseau, 2018: 26).

13. The use of faithful witnessing represents acts of resistance; Yomaira C. Figueroa-Vásquez describes "faithful witnessing as a lens through which to recognize the assertion of humanity and dignity in moments when these would otherwise be unseen or ignored . . . Without

Another significant cultural influence in Guyana can be attributed to the Asian indentured laborers, both Indian and Chinese. Following the abolition of slavery in Guyana in 1834, British colonists recognized the region's profitability for the continued extraction of resources such as rice and sugar. In the ensuing eighty-year period, they instituted a distinct labor system called indentureship (Hardwick 2014, 1). During this era, a substantial number of Indians and a smaller contingent of Chinese people were brought to Guyana under contractual arrangements spanning three to seven years, with the understanding that they could return to their countries of origin upon completing their terms (Bahadur 2013, 77).

Nevertheless, many Indian indentured laborers opted to remain in Guyana and establish their lives in this new land with the promise of receiving property (Sen 2009, 68–69). Unfortunately, this process of hard labor and exploitation denied the Indians many aspects of their culture, such as language, religion, epistemologies, food, and values. The most enduring cultural legacy of the Indian heritage in Guyana is found in its food culture. Like the displaced Amerindians and enslaved Africans, traces of Indian cuisine endured, ultimately playing an essential role in the constitution of Guyanese cuisine. In Guyana, the Indo-Guyanese mark of the culinary tradition is salient, with the preservation and adaptation of curries. Alongside roti, it showcases the richness of Indian spices and culinary traditions, seamlessly integrated into the broader Guyanese culinary landscape. This culinary achievement underscores the remarkable ability to adapt and evolve within a new geographical context and to incorporate novel ingredients into a *standard dish* (Richards-Greaves 2013, 87–88; Sen 2009, 73–74). Curry encompasses various interpretations. Colleen Taylor Sen's definition resonates most with the colonial history of Guyana. She describes curry as a spiced stew of meat, fish, or vegetables, typically served with rice, bread, or another starch. This dish, whether wet or dry, is flavored with curry powder—a blend of spices like turmeric, cumin seed, coriander seed, chilies, and fenugreek—originating from British India in the late eighteenth century. In India, curry encompasses many dishes like

this kind of recognition, histories are erased, silenced, and ultimately invalidated as human experiences" (Figueroa-Vásquez 2020, 70–71).

korma, *rogan josh*, *molee*, *vindaloo*, and *doh piaza*, reflecting the diverse culinary landscape. However, these diverse dishes were condensed into a singular cooking style in the Guyanese context, utilizing locally available ingredients and imported curry powder blends (Sen 2009, 7–14).

The creolization of Indo-Guyanese curry further enriches its flavors, blending influences from India, the Caribbean, and the diverse ethnic groups within Guyana.[14] Adapting local ingredients, such as fish, plantains, and cassava, into traditional Indian dishes resulted in a unique culinary tradition. For instance, Indo-Guyanese curry distinguishes itself by adding allspice and coconut milk, which produces a sweet and spicy flavor profile. Moreover, noticeable differences emerged in the preparation and taste of Indo-Guyanese dishes compared to their Indian counterparts; for one, it is less spicy. Guyanese curry has also sparked debates within the

---

14. Creolization emerges as a dynamic process, weaving diverse influences to shape hybrid cultures and identities. Guyana, renowned for its vibrant cultural diversity, exemplifies this phenomenon vividly, particularly in its culinary landscape (Garth 2013, 5). While creolization is often discussed in linguistic contexts; its impact extends deeply into gastronomy, reflecting a fusion of traditions from various ethnic groups.

The term "creole" traces back centuries, with roots in colonial Peru, where individuals born in the region but disconnected from their European heritage were labeled as such. Over time, Creoles evolved into a distinct cultural group, often opposing colonial powers due to their unfamiliarity with dominant customs (Collier and Fleischmann 2003, xv). Ethnicity initially played a minor role in defining Creoles, but racial distinctions emerged, particularly in plantation colonies, where skin color became a defining factor. Fernando Ortiz introduced the concept of transculturation, emphasizing cultural transformation by introducing new elements and creating entirely new cultural phenomena. While similar to creolization, some scholars argue that transculturation may overlook demographic differences (Chomsky et al. 2019, 26–27). However, creolization offers a more nuanced understanding of cultural exchange, particularly in Guyana's culinary scene. In Guyana, creolization manifests in a tantalizing blend of culinary traditions from Amerindian, Chinese, Indo-Guyanese, Afro-Guyanese, and European groups. This fusion celebrates the diversity of Guyanese heritage while preserving the individuality of each culture. Rather than a mere melting pot, Guyana's cuisine represents a masterful blend that underscores the enduring influence of creolization on the nation's culinary identity. In essence, creolization is a central force shaping Guyana's culinary landscape, uniting diverse influences to create a multifaceted culinary flavor. It celebrates the richness of each culture while embracing the transformative power of cultural exchange, resulting in a culinary experience that is both enticing and deeply rooted in Guyanese heritage.

Caribbean, such as the linguistic preference for "Chicken Curry" or "Curry Chicken" (Thompson 2021). These adaptations and innovations in Indo-Guyanese cuisine showcase the cultural exchange and creativity stemming from colonial history and diversity. The resulting culinary experience is both familiar and refreshingly unique, embodying Guyana's cultural heritage we know today.

Colonial history destroyed the sense of identity for those in the diaspora, and the dominant culture collapsed our identity into a singular definition. Even though Indo-Guyanese people are from different parts of India with different languages and cultural practices, all were reduced to workers in the plantations and then named Indians as a way of erasing differences.[15] This reduces the diversity of experiences into one notion, which becomes the marker for who they are by being named by the dominant Western voices. Edward Said describes this as *orientalism* (Said 1979). Similarly, we see this in the transformation of Indian cuisine in the anglophone Caribbean and Guyana; the definition of *curry* for us in Guyana is any dish, wet or dry, flavored with curry powder. Even though historically there was no singular definition for curry in the subcontinent, the British colonial capture of this dish transformed it into the singular description that we use in Guyana and other parts of the anglophone Caribbean.

Despite their relatively small population in Guyana (0.18 percent of the population: Bureau of Statistics 2016, 5), the Chinese have also had a notable influence on the country's culinary landscape. Colloquially referred to as "Chinese food," this cuisine has become a distinctive and integral element of the Guyanese culinary tradition, imparting unique Chinese flavors and cooking techniques. Cynthia Nelson, a Guyanese chef, wants Chinese food to become Guyana's national dish because of its recognizability and distinctive flavors in Guyanese culture (Nelson 2010, 81–83).

---

15. In the ongoing narrative of reclaiming identity, the term "coolie" has undergone a transformation from a pejorative label to a badge of honor for some Indo-Guyanese. Among these trailblazers are Rajkumari Singh, a celebrated poet from Guyana, and Gaiutra Bahadur, a renowned writer whose roots trace back to Bihar, India. Their efforts have been pivotal in reshaping the perception of "coolie" from one of shame to pride (Kumar 2017, xiv–xv).

The Chinese culinary influences are unmistakably present through dishes such as chow mien and fried rice, reflecting the art of aromatic stir-frying and inventive flavor combinations. Chinese cuisine has become an integral part of Guyanese culinary tradition, representing a successful fusion of Chinese culinary elements with Guyanese preferences.

Many Guyanese academics and activists have advocated for the relegation of colonization to the annals of history and a collective focus on the future (Henry 2019). Nonetheless, the contemporary sociopolitical framework in Guyana reveals that while the overt manifestations of colonization—characterized by the horrors of enslavement and forced plantation labor—have faded, more sophisticated mechanisms of control and power persist. During my participation in a Diasporic Conference at the University of Guyana during the spring of 2023, tensions escalated when discussions delved into the enduring legacy of colonization and the persistent issues of anti-Blackness within Guyanese communities. The traumatic responses and impassioned outbursts from attendees underscored that the historical trauma stemming from this violence continues to resonate within the collective consciousness and bodies of the Guyanese populace.

Guyana's declaration of independence on May 26, 1966, did not signify the cessation of colonization rooted in domination and control. Instead, it marked the onset of a new phase of neocolonization, albeit under the guise of national autonomy. It was during this period that the prominence of racial and class divisions became further entrenched, with Guyana's national elections, even to this day, being determined along racial lines (Misir 2010, 29–31). In the years following independence, Guyana, under the dictatorial leadership of Linden Forbes Burnham, was mandated to "produce or perish." This represented yet another dark chapter in the arduous journey of the Guyanese community as they navigated the complexities of survival within this environment (Richards-Greaves 2013, 77).

Guyana's cultural evolution is one of resilience, adaptation, and resistance. Centuries ago, European colonizers arrived, driven by a quest for resources and cheap labor. Their presence reshaped Guyana's landscape and society, disrupting Indigenous communities and enslaving Africans. Despite this upheaval, Guyana's diverse peoples showed remarkable resilience, preserving and adapting their cultural traditions amidst the violence. Out of this tumult emerged creolization. Indigenous, African, Indian, and Chinese communities interacted, blending their customs, languages, and cuisines to create a creolized identity. Creolization became a form of survival and resistance, allowing these marginalized groups to assert their agency within the confines of colonial domination.

Today, globalization shapes Guyana's cultural landscape. While offering opportunities for connectivity and exchange, globalization also poses challenges. Local traditions risk being overshadowed by global homogenization, threatening heritage preservation. However, the Guyanese people persist in seeking cultural autonomy and self-determination. Guyanese communities navigate the complexities of the modern world with resilience and determination while honoring the past. In doing so, we forge a path that embraces tradition and innovation, ensuring that our cultural legacy endures for generations to come.

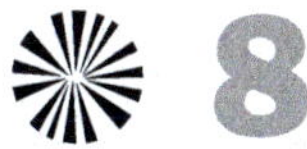 8

Revolutionizing Democracy, Contravening (Non)Human Rights

Food Insecurity in Plurinational Ecuador and Bolivia

Steven James

IN PLURINATIONALISM, food insecurity is less about utilizing certain types of food to assail disenfranchised groups; rather, it stems from piecemeal solutions to ecological and racial injustices in the history and contemporary politics of the state.[1] Since returning to democracy, Ecuador (1979) and Bolivia (1982) have allowed food insecurity to disproportionately impact marginalized cultural and ethnic groups, including Indigenous and Afro-descendant peoples. Ecuador and Bolivia—the only two countries in the world to proclaim a plurinational identity in their constitutions—consider themselves democratic. They revolutionized their definitions of democracy—Ecuador in 2008 and Bolivia in 2009—to explicitly include

1. I am a cisgender, queer, white man from Dallas. I became interested in the topic of plurinationalism, including how it shapes food sovereignty and racialized peoples' civil rights more broadly, from my ministerial work in Dallas and traveling in Latin America for ethnographic research. I acknowledge that, despite having gained expertise on plurinationalism, my positionality may make me miss critical dynamics.

food sovereignty[2] for disenfranchised groups, in addition to protecting nonhuman animals and the environment to advance ecological justice and sustainability. However, Ecuador and Bolivia actively contravene food sovereignty. They prevent disenfranchised groups from fighting their own hunger and force these groups to feed those who already have access to healthy, safe, and sustainable agricultural and food systems. Food sovereignty should protect disenfranchised groups from exploitation and annihilation, but their current treatment in plurinational Ecuador and Bolivia makes these groups expendable.

THE HISTORY OF PLURINATIONALISM AND CONSTITUTIONAL RIGHTS IN ECUADOR AND BOLIVIA

In the 1970s and 1980s, when Ecuador, Bolivia, and other Andean countries transitioned from military to civilian rule, "the Native Andean people joined social movement organizations that opened up new opportunities for them to influence national legislative agendas," including granting the environment rights, making food sovereignty a basic human right, and eventually transitioning to plurinationalism (Marín-Dale 2016, 260). Plurinationalism is a postcolonial form of government that seeks to break ties with colonial legacies and encourages representation and rights for marginalized communities, "[proposing] a new model of state in the institutional, cultural, economic, democratic, territorial, and administration of justice areas" (Salazar 2022, 182). It is a form of representative democracy. Indigenous ecologies represent deep-rooted ecological wisdom, such as traditional ecological knowledge (TEK) and communal management of natural resources, which represent a harmonious relationship between humans and Nature. These perspectives are inherent to cultural traditions, agency, and survival. Ethno-territorial rights, self-determination, and

2. Food sovereignty is the right for cultural and ethnic groups to practice their own agricultural and food systems, sustainably producing culturally appropriate and healthy food. Plurinationalism in Ecuador and Bolivia also grants the environment constitutional rights, Indigenous people land sovereignty, and Afro-descendant and other cultural and ethnic groups antiracist safeguards. Ecuador 2008 (rev. 2021) Constitution, Articles 15, 281; and "Food Sovereignty," U.S. Food Sovereignty Alliance, October 2023, https://usfoodsovereigntyalliance.org/what-is-food-sovereignty/.

environmental policymaking (e.g., *Sumak Kawsay* [Kichwa "good living"; Spanish *buen vivir*] in Ecuador's Constitution, or *Suma Qamaña* [Aymara "live well"; Spanish *vivir bien*] in Bolivia's Constitution) exemplify the implementation of Indigenous ecologies into the wider practices of a plurinational state.

Plurinationalism in Ecuador and Bolivia treats nature as a vibrant entity, known as Pachamama (Mother Earth).[3] The land, under the concept of "good living"/"live well," holds special meaning not only to Indigenous peoples, but to the country as a whole. The move to plurinationalism in Ecuador and Bolivia involved the codification of Pachamama as living and worthy of value. If Pachamama "has inherent value and is interconnected, interdependent, interrelated, then the fulfillment of nonmaterial and material needs can only be achieved through everyday practices and ethical principles that seek to co-exist in a harmonious and balanced way with the community of nature and all other communities of the world" (Dolhare and Rojas-Lizana 2017, 21). Considering Pachamama worthy of rights involves fighting poverty, eradicating climate change, creating opportunities for persecuted communities, and securing the well-being and potential of future generations. This progress included the addition of *Sumak Kawsay/buen vivir* to the 2008 Ecuadorian Constitution and *Suma Qamaña/vivir bien* to the 2009 Bolivian Constitution.

Ecuador's 2008 Constitution considers food sovereignty one of the basic principles of the state. Bolivia's 2009 Constitution also guarantees "[food] sovereignty for the entire population."[4]

Food sovereignty in plurinationalism has co-opted Indigenous perspectives of nature. The concept of "good living"/"live well"—the results of Indigenous social movements—claims that humanity not only benefits from a relationship with nature (or the Supreme Being Pachamama), but is also a part of nature.[5] This notion of relationality with Pachamama influenced Ecuadorian and Bolivian politicians and activists to give nature constitutional rights. However, despite the codification of food sover-

3. From the Andean Quechua language.

4. Bolivia (Plurinational State of) 2009 Constitution, Article 255.

5. Ecuador 2008 Constitution and Bolivia 2009 Constitution.

eignty, agrarian and food systems have not considerably improved for disenfranchised groups (McKay, Nehring, and Walsh-Dilley 2014, 1177; Tilzey 2018, 275). In Ecuador, food sovereignty is "focused on increasing the productivity and efficiency of small- and medium-sized producers conceived as private farmers along capitalist lines" (Henderson 2017, 45), and in Bolivia, "racist ideologies persist that maintain class hierarchies associating peasants with the lower stratum of society" (Mercado and Hjortsø 2023, 2). Both the Indigenous and non-Indigenous government authorities, such as President Rafael Correa of Ecuador (2007–2017) and President Evo Morales of Bolivia (2006–2019) (the former being a *mestizo* who ran on a platform of Indigenous support, and the latter being Indigenous Aymara who advocated for his community and became his country's first Indigenous president) continue to co-opt, and speak for, Indigenous peoples who do not have access to the privilege of government authority, "[feeling] pressure to accommodate to these ideologies [such as systemic racism] because they claim to question discrimination and include non-whites" (Martínez Novo 2018, 395).

FOOD INSECURITY: STATISTICS

Indigenous peoples in Ecuador and Bolivia are put in a position to feed the country when they cannot provide for themselves. Rural households in Ecuador and Bolivia rely on what they grow themselves for food. Most people in rural communities own small plots and go hungry in lean seasons.[6] Those who live in rural Bolivian households, such as children and working adults, are nutritionally stunted compared to those who live in urban areas. In plurinational Ecuador and Bolivia, the data, normally collected by interest groups, academics, NGOs, and aid-based organizations, do not always reflect marginal lived experiences. Furthermore, constitutional rights to food sovereignty (and land protection) are rarely enforced.[7]

---

6. Times throughout the year when food prices rise and jobs are in short supply.

7. The 2022 Global Hunger Index (GHI) ranks Ecuador 70th out of 121, with a score of 15.2, meaning that Ecuador has moderate food security. See "Global Hunger Index 2023: Ecuador," *Global Hunger Index*: https://www.globalhungerindex.org/ecuador.html. Similarly, Bolivia ranks 61st, with a score of 13.2, also indicating moderate food security. "Bolivia (Plurinational State of)," *Global Hunger Index*: https://www.globalhungerindex.org/bolivia.html.

In Ecuador, poverty rates decreased between 2021 and 2022 from 28 to 25 percent alongside a 3 percent rise in GDP (United Nations World Food Program, "Ecuador: Annual Country Report" 2022, 9). Furthermore, Ecuador has the second-highest rate of chronic mild nutrition in the region (after Guatemala), at 27 percent for the overall population and 30 percent in rural areas. In May 2022, 61 percent of migrants had jobs, but only 21 percent held formal employment. Due to climate change, droughts, earthquakes, volcanic activity, landslides, and floods have increased since 2014, contributing not only to food insecurity, but also loss of life and home. Nearly nine hundred thousand tons of food in Ecuador is lost or wasted annually, according to the Harvard Law School Food Law and Policy Clinic and the Global FoodBanking Network's *The Global Food Donation Policy Atlas*, which tracks food security laws and policies globally. Approximately 33 percent of the population experienced food insecurity between 2018 and 2020, according to the Atlas, a near-threefold increase from 2014 to 2016.[8]

In addition to increased natural disasters from climate change, food produced and consumed near mines and landfills also contributes to the chronic child malnutrition spreading throughout rural areas. Even though in 2022 Ecuador passed the Law to Prevent and Reduce Food Loss and Waste and Reduce the Hunger of People in Vulnerable Situations, also known as the "FLW Law," to address food loss and waste within the supply chain and to encourage donations of safe and nutritional food, contaminated soil and water from development projects infect the crustaceans ($5.33 billion USD of the country's annual exports in 2022), bananas ($3.76 billion), and processed fish ($1.27 billion) that go to the United States, China, Panama, Chile, and Russia. Ecuador is one of the world's largest exporters of crustaceans and bananas, and recent developments, such as the intervention of the United States as a major actor in Ecuadorian food politics, could mean that *campesinos*[9] will continue to grow less for themselves and more for the people who exploit them. Furthermore, widespread protests in June 2022 caused $9 million USD in damages to the

8. See Harvard Law School Food Law and Policy Clinic and the Global FoodBanking Network, *The Global Food Donation Policy Atlas*, 2023: https://atlas.foodbanking.org/.

9. Spanish for "[peasant] farmers," normally an Indigenous person.

country's shrimp industry, according to National Chamber of Aquaculture Executive President José Antonio Camposano. At that time, the Confederation of Indigenous Nationalities of Ecuador (CONAIE), the country's largest Indigenous organization (representing more than 70 percent, or at least 770,000 of the country's Indigenous people) led protests in response to increasing oil and food prices and increased mining activity under the economic policies of President Guillermo Lasso. The protests turned violent and led to road blockades, preventing supplies from reaching different parts of the country.

The Bolivian government has committed to ending extreme poverty by 2025 and international organizations such as the United Nations World Food Program (WFP) have committed to supporting local initiatives to help alleviate these issues. "Smallholder farmers contribute significantly to Bolivia's food production system, yet they are also among the most vulnerable to food insecurity and malnutrition, especially Indigenous people in rural areas where 30 percent live in poverty," with children facing historic levels of malnutrition and women encountering dangerous levels of gender-based violence (United Nations World Food Program, "Plurinational State of Bolivia: Annual Country Report" 2022, 18). The WFP and other international organizations, as well as federal governments including Germany, have helped "provide food assistance to crisis-affected populations, resilience building, support smallholder farmers, and institutional strengthening" (WFP 2022, 10).

The nutritional stunting rate for Bolivian children under five for the general population dropped from 33 to 16 percent in that same time, though in rural areas, where Indigenous peoples tend to live, the rate is 23.7 percent (WFP 2022,10). While people in cities tend to eat meat and other foods that help them gain weight, the staple of Indigenous peoples such as the Quechua, Aymara, and Guarani in rural areas tend to include potatoes, rice, maize, legumes, and soybeans. Soybean meal is one of the country's chief exports (720 million US dollars, only to be exceeded by natural resources),[10] and *campesinos* must travel to sell their crops in the

10. "Bolivia," Observatory of Economic Complexity, 2023, https://oec.world/en/profile/country/bol.

market and to the government to help feed their families and communities. In 2022, the total number of food-insecure people was 6.3 million, or slightly more than half of the country's population, with 25 percent of this part of the population facing severe food insecurity (WFP 2022, 8). Women are 26 percent less likely than men to work, a view "primarily explained by gendered and social norms that view domestic and unpaid care work as the responsibility of women" (WFP 2022, 21). Furthermore, approximately 40 percent of women live in poverty, and they tend to have less access to education and land tenure, and fewer assets than men.

While agricultural exports drive economic leverage in the region, "food insecurity remains a daily reality for millions of Latin Americans" (Adams 2020, 54). Bolivia is one of Latin America and the Caribbean's poorest countries, particularly in rural areas, with the highest level of undernourishment in South America. Many Bolivian households cannot afford the minimum nutritional intake for healthy living, nor do they have regular access to food. Those in rural areas can also fall victim to being nutritionally stunted, a problem that disproportionately impacts children and women. Approximately two-thirds of Bolivia's Indigenous population also lives among 50 percent of the country's poor (Andersen 2010, 94). However, because they are Indigenous, they are automatically treated as nonhuman. The government non-consensually ties their being to the land, irascibly intervening in their lives to ruin any hope their people have of a future beyond extinction. For the South American Indigenous peoples with whom I have spoken, they fear this means soon.

While it is easy to assume this only affects people in rural areas, Santa Cruz, Bolivia's largest city (with four million inhabitants) and producer of more than half of the country's food, must also ration its water and has noticed a decline in food production and export. Rainfall has decreased by 26 percent in Santa Cruz between 2022 and 2023, according to the *Instituto Nacional de Estadística*.[11] Sometimes, protests are so intense that Bolivia shuts down food exports, including beef and soybean flour. This

11. "*Bolivia—Temperatura Media por Ciudades, Según Año y Mes, 1990–2023*," Instituto Nacional de Estadística, December 2023, https://www.ine.gob.bo/index.php/medio-ambiente/clima-y-atmosfera/.

poses a threat to the country's disenfranchised groups, which not only means racial/ethnic minorities, but also undocumented migrants—mostly from Venezuela and Colombia, becoming the Latin American country to receive the largest number of migrants in general in recent years—and the persisting impacts of the COVID-19 pandemic.

ANDEAN THEOLOGIES: ECOLOGICAL AND RACIAL INJUSTICES

(Non)humans in Ecuador and Bolivia have combined hybrid religiosity, liberation theology, and decolonial social ethics, emphasizing "the relationships between heaven, nature, and human beings . . . and [the fact that] there is no severance of the unit of the profane and the sacred" (de la Torre and Eloisa 2016, 481). Some of these cosmologies, which have converged with Catholicism, have "provided a vehicle for the cultural resistance of indigenous peoples and for the political mobilization of the rural and urban working classes" (475). They "provide an important site for civic engagement, moral synthesis, and for building bonds of solidarity and cohesion" (Walsh-Dilley 2019, 501). Furthermore, many Christians in Ecuador and most in Bolivia are Indigenous, meaning Christianity is an inherent part of their Indigenous identities, including their languages, cosmovisions, and fights for cultural survival.

Andean theologies, such as those in Ecuador and Bolivia, do not separate Christianity from Indigenous or even Afro-descendant cosmologies. They promote sociobiocentric interrelationality and recognize that different forms of life require emotional and spiritual care and intertwined relationships in "good living" (and "live well") (Hoskins 2023, 17–18). The primary practitioners and leaders in these theologies are not clergy, but rather the laity who depend on the sharing of food, work, political engagement, and living on and connecting with the land. They combine traditional tenets of Catholic theology such as life and dignity of the human person, the freedom and empowerment of liberation theology, the collective well-being of *Sumak Kawsay/buen vivir/Suma Qamaña/vivir bien*, and to a lesser extent the scriptural authority of the region's increasingly present evangelical communities. Theologies autochthonous to the Andes defy neoliberal standards of individualism, privatization, competition, deregulation, and free market capitalism that afflict promoting food security. Furthermore, Ecuadorian and

Bolivian *campesinos* are not always paid their fair share for their labor. Cheap food is available in the United States and other Western countries due to "the destruction of peasant, indigenous, and other livelihoods, and a racialized and gendered division of global labor" (Dunford 2017, 387). Less and less does income goes to those who produce the food, and workers have begun to feel the sting of economic inequality, a reduction of public services and international aid, becoming their country's scapegoats, and social unrest.

Furthermore, theological perspectives in the past decade, within Ecuador and Bolivia and internationally, have been shaped around concerns of Indigenous peoples to normalize the ethics of caring nationally and globally for the (non)human and align it with the prioritization of caring for the poor and vulnerable, solidarity, and other themes of Catholic social teaching (Pope Paul VI 1965, I.1–2.9). Some of this comes from Pope Francis, who has critiqued the neoliberalism, overconsumption, and effects of climate change that have made disenfranchised populations, including Indigenous and Afro-descendant peoples, even more vulnerable, calling on fellow Catholics to do the same. While he does not offer a practical way to approach these forms of oppressive suffering, Francis recognizes that pressure is put on these communities "to abandon their homelands to make room for agricultural or mining projects which are undertaken without regard for the degradation of nature and culture" (Pope Francis 2015, IV.2.146).[12]

The theologies of Indigenous Christians also engage that which decolonial thought in the academy often disregards: the refusal to speak for Indigenous and instead speak with Indigenous people on their terms. This helps to make theoretical contributions less essentialized and more self-critical, while also living up to decoloniality's promise to tear down Western mores that excuse natural resource extraction, militarism, political control, economic leverage, and epistemic and physical genocide (Martínez

12. *Laudato Si'* addresses the whole world. Jorge Mario Bergoglio (now Pope Francis) chose the name Francis after St. Francis of Assisi, the patron saint of animals and the environment. He calls for nongovernmental organizations, social movements, and fellow Catholics to protect the lands of Afro-descendant, Indigenous, and other populations by pressuring national governments to enact and practice legislation that protects both environmental and human rights, but that is the extent of his praxis in the document.

Novo 2018, 390, 410; Mignolo 2020, 616). Onto-epistemic hierarchies normalize the idea that those on the underside of (postcolonial) history develop ecological proposals contextually, with Euro-American mores under modernity/coloniality applicable globally. Pushing back means paying attention to what happens at the grassroots level while also reflecting and developing a praxis at hyperlocal and international levels. The cosmopolitanism of modernity/coloniality refuses to pay attention to the perspectives of those on its underside, and when it does it essentializes the poor and oppressed as (non)human subjects of study. Given that the onto-epistemologies of Andean theologies emerged in Latin America as a result of Indigenous Christians embracing their inherent contradictions and multiplicities, not "in Europe as a development of French critical radicalism in passage from the structuralist episteme to the nascent ecological episteme," they conflict with and contradict those of modernity/coloniality (Leff 2012, 8). Because "social injustice in the modern capitalist era has everything to do with the equation of much of humanity with Nature, regarded as a realm to be exploited and appropriated in the process of accumulating capital," humanity must overcome its fear of nature and the nonhuman to embrace that which it deems less than (Fisher 2019, 148).

Unlike Euro-American Christianity, which constructs a hierarchy that places humanity over the rest of creation, the Indigenous peoples of Ecuador and Bolivia take a decolonial approach to existing in relationship with the rest of creation. Unfortunately, these countries' preference for Euro-American Christianity over Indigenous cosmologies necessitates the involvement of church actors into peace negotiations, with oppressively violent situations repeating the cycles of extractive capitalism and settler colonialism.

In Ecuador and Bolivia, when the government cannot provide for its citizens, social unrest occurs. In June 2022, in Ecuador, when protestors combatted rises in food prices, led by CONAIE, they blocked roads that Indigenous peoples need for food and grain. Bishop Rafael Cob shared that "it is clear that the current Ecuadorian administration has a neoliberal nature, and that has an impact on the lives of the working poor."[13] Indigenous

13. Eduardo Campos Lima, "In Ecuador, Catholic Bishops Help Negotiate End to Massive Protests," *National Catholic Reporter*, August 1, 2022.

activists demanded that the drilling on ancestral lands must stop. The drilling contaminated the soil and water necessary to produce agriculture and for Indigenous peoples to exercise their relationality with nature. The road-blocking caused some people to starve, with farmers lacking access to the routes they needed to arrive at the market. Social unrest is also a consequence of antidecolonial sentiment, such as what has happened recently in Bolivia. In November 2019, following a US-backed coup, government official Luis Fernando Camacho knelt before a Bible and the country's flag, proclaiming: "Bolivia for Christ, Pachamama will never again enter [the presidential] palace."[14] This led to more social unrest, causing Indigenous protestors to block trade routes farmers used to transport food and grain. Father Osvaldo Chirveches shared that the church hesitated to end the blockades because of its alleged role in removing Evo Morales from office.

NATURE, GENDER, AND COMMODIFICATION

The negative treatment of nature coincides with that of gender, as "the Western colonial, modern, capitalist structuring of the construction of social life, the production of knowledge included, is saturated with racialized gender meanings and gives form to particular, historical systems of racialized gender formation," maintaining the view that women are caretakers and that their bodies exist merely to reproduce (Lugones 2020, 36). The construction and treatment of gender belong to the (plurinational) state, for "[t]he concept of gender itself carries conceptual, social, metaphysical, historical meaning that is inimical to the on-the-ground resistance by the inhabitants of *Abya Yala*,"[15] even when it also allows for their destruction (36). Furthermore, gendered and sexualized violence has yet to become an inherent part of decolonial thought (36). A further examination of their multiple encounters with plurinational power dynamics as subjects and citizens could help decolonial activists and intellectuals further the dialogue about the lack of the treatment of gender in decoloniality and decolonization (Femenías 2020, 45).

14. Idem., "Bolivian Catholic Church Cautious About Addressing Recent Social Unrest," *National Catholic Reporter*, December 12, 2022.

15. The Kula term for "vital blood," meaning "the Americas."

The empowerment of girls and women has become central to sustaining food security in Ecuador and Bolivia. Violence against girls and women remains a systemic issue in both countries, with girls and women calling for the deconstruction of gender stereotypes and accessibility to participating in decision-making processes at the local and national levels. One way they have done this is by leading the way in sustainable agricultural production, slowly increasing their autonomy over their bodies and land rights. *Campesinas*, and women in general, are forced to find creative and resilient ways to produce food for their families and communities amid food insecurity. Sustainable Agriculture with Gender Inclusion and Participation, a program in Quito, Ecuador[16] that trains female-headed households and women in agro-ecology, technology, and food accessibility, so far has had fifty-six thousand urban farmers participate (nearly 86 percent of which are women); some have started their own sustainable gardens.[17] The program addresses social justice concerns, such as the fact that "[p]eople who live in Quito, women in particular, have limited access to formal education and employment" beyond agriculture.[18] Women in Ecuador, especially Indigenous women, tend to lack access to schooling and employment, so the project helps female-headed households learn to grow crops, fruits, medicinal and ornamental plants, and vegetables for personal consumption and selling. Much of Bolivia's food security is organized by women, who perceive food insecurity as a form of violence that targets marginalized communities. For the past decade, national and international actors in Bolivia have attempted to engage with women in decision-making, with NGOs such as Global Exchange on a Transformative Advocacy Exchange financing farming projects that specifically recruit women.

However, Indigenous land claims such as those of the Kichwa and Tsáchila remain secondary to the concerns of the government, and when

---

16. The country's capital.

17. United Nations Framework Convention on Climate Change, "Sustainable Agriculture with Gender Inclusion and Participation—Ecuador," 2023, https://unfccc.int/climate-action/momentum-for-change/women-for-results/sustainable-agriculture-with-gender-inclusion-and-participation-ecuador.

18. United Nations Framework Convention on Climate Change, "Sustainable Agriculture."

it comes to Indigenous women, their relationship with the land is normally shaped by highly racialized, gendered, and sexualized cultural, economic, and political interests to which they do not consent. Unlike men, who normally have the means to find other work and rule the household, Indigenous Ecuadorian women's relationships with land is one of feeding the local community and their families—in other words, caregiving—which the government exploits. Fully aware that Indigenous women tend to have less access to agricultural land (and land in general) compared to men and are more likely to rent land for agricultural production, the government forces women to articulate gender-specific discourses, such as being a *female* head of house, a situation that was normalized by the lack of concerns articulated specific to women when the country was becoming plurinational (Radcliffe 2014, 857). Furthermore, "[t]he lack of systematic attention to women's land rights—whether as individuals or members of ethnic collectives—was furthered under the 2008 Constitution," granting ethno-territorial rights and political autonomy for Indigenous and Afro-descendant populations, but leaving gender and sexual concerns about these rights to the mercy of local elections, which are normally dominated by men (859). For women—and, I would add, anybody who is not a cisgender male—ethno-territorial reforms impede rights; they do not advance them (860). Furthermore, with the exclusion of women, it is impossible for a community to collectively decide how to combat land-related issues, such as systematic agricultural and food development.

Furthermore, modernity/coloniality puts Indigenous women in rigid binaries based on concepts of gender. In "the post-structural feminism perspective, gender is constructed in connection with the society and the culture . . . and self-employment will continue to play a critical role in enabling women to participate in economic activity, particularly for women in rural areas or cultures, such as those in most indigenous communities" (Padilla-Meléndez 2022, 855). Indigenous women in Bolivia enact entrepreneurship, resilience, and sustainability in their communities to prevent climate-related and nutritional shocks in their communities. The notion that women are caretakers has also extended to relationships with Pachamama. Ecuadorian and Bolivian politics portray "her" as a vibrant but static entity whose sole purpose—like those of Indigenous peoples (especially women)—is to provide humans with food, natural resources, and other means of neoliberal overconsumption.

The thingification of Pachamama in Ecuadorian and Bolivian politics and constitutionalism—and of women—shaped by misplaced notions of gender and "good living"/"live well," not only excludes from decision-making Andean and Amazonian peoples who do not connect with the Supreme Being but will continue the cycle of this metaphysical and epistemic violence in plurinational food security. "Throughout Western modernity, the relation between nature and society has been organized around a rigid binary in which the earth constitutes the feminized and racialized backdrop for human endeavors," turning the Earth into a rigid, gendered, and colonized subject (Tola 2018, 28). Women—particularly Indigenous women—and nature are sexualized in such a way that those in power view them as commodities.

CONCLUSION

Ecuador and Bolivia have failed to implement food sovereignty, which could have provided disenfranchised groups the freedom and security necessary to ensure systematic agricultural and food development (Peña 2013, 6). Forced politicization of racialized and sexualized groups contravenes their civil rights. Revolutionizing democracy, in the form of plurinationalism, must do more than codify food sovereignty; it must also safeguard disenfranchised groups from threats to their cosmologies and their survival.

SECTION III

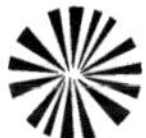

AFRICA

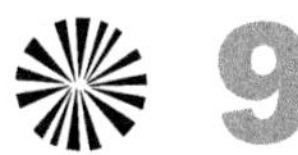 9

Food as a Weapon

The Case of Gwata Village in Zimbabwe's Mutasa District

Terence Mupangwa

ZIMBABWE HAS BEEN HIT with high levels of unemployment and poverty. Since 2000, the economy of Zimbabwe has been in decline. Between January and July 2008, inflation escalated at an alarming rate of 250,000,000 percent (Hanke and Kwok 2009, 355). The Zimbabwe Vulnerability Assessment Committee (ZIMVAC) (2019) records that 7.7 million Zimbabweans were food insecure in 2019: 5.5 million in rural areas and 2.2 million in urban areas. In 2020, the food security situation got worse and 8.8 million both in urban and rural areas were having problems with securing food (Moyo 2022). The general indication is that the rural population are the most affected in terms of food security. A number of reasons have been given to explain this state of affairs. Amongst them is the fast-track land program in which farms were taken from the white farmers and given to Indigenous farmers from the year 2000 onwards. According to Moyo (2022), most farmers have not been able to produce enough maize; for instance, in 2019 they managed to produce 777,000 tons compared with a national requirement of 1.4 million tons. In 2020, there was a slight increase to 908,000 tons but the country still recorded a deficit. Such deficits of the staple crop translate into limited access to food for many, especially the rural folk. However, there are some farmers who are capable of producing a good amount of maize, who have technical expertise and experience but are being affected by the economic situation of the country. The economy of the country currently is characterized by high inflation rates, a weak currency, and high national debt. Funding and credit for farming are scarce, leading to subpar production from farmers despite their expertise and experience. Additionally, climatic changes have led to food shortages in Zimbabwe. The country has been experiencing droughts, prolonged mid-season dry spells, floods, and cyclones. Besides negatively affecting crop production, climatic changes also have a huge negative impact on livestock production, which is a critical component of the country's food system. The province of Matabeleland, which is the country's major producer of livestock, lost thousands of livestock in 2019 and 2020 (Dube-Matutu 2020; Mpofu 2019). The COVID-19 pandemic exacerbated the situation in 2020, since people were supposed to be staying at home. Very little was done in terms of food production during the pandemic. Hence, it is not surprising that the country is experiencing acute food shortages. Since the country has failed to produce enough food, many, especially in rural areas, need help to survive. Given this context, the research conducted for this chapter sought to ascertain how the Zimbabwean government is using food as a weapon to exert control over the villagers in Gwata village.

POLITICAL CONTEXT

Since Zimbabwe gained independence in 1980, the ruling Zimbabwe African National Union – Patriotic Front (ZANU-PF) party has been in power. They faced no serious political opposition until 1999, when the Movement for Democratic Change (MDC) was formed, which ushered in a significant shift in Zimbabwean politics (Makonye 2021). MDC was organized under the leadership of Morgan Tsvangirai to challenge President Robert Mugabe's ZANU-PF. Since then, the MDC has undergone a series of splits and reorganizations. The most prominent splinter party has been the Citizens Coalition for Change (CCC or Triple C), which has since remained a formidable opposition party. In 2000, when the Zimbabwean government realized that it was losing ground, especially in urban areas, it sought to regain support by implementing a program to take land from white farmers and give it to black Zimbabweans (Madimu 2020). This program was not well planned and was executed haphazardly. Its poor planning affected food production in the country in a negative way (Runganga, Njoroge and Mishi 2022; Madimu 2020). Most of the people who took over the farms had no knowledge of commercial food production. This led to the reduction of food in the country (Madimu 2020). As the years went by, food became scarcer as the political terrain became more volatile and the new farmers failed to produce enough food for the country. On the political side, Tsvangirai, the president of the opposition party MDC, defeated Robert Mugabe in the presidential election of 2008. Though Mugabe was beaten, Morgan Tsvangirai did not acquire enough votes as stipulated by the country's constitution to be the president. This led to a rerun of the presidential election. The announcement of the rerun led to a shift towards political violence, which ultimately killed more than two hundred activists, mainly from the MDC (Chitando and Togarasei 2010). The subsequent political instability impacted the country's economy. The political environment has led to Western sanctions. Zimbabwean politics in essence scared investors from doing business in the country. Industries and companies closed, worsening the food crisis (Mlambo 2017).

TRADITIONAL AGRICULTURE IN GWATA VILLAGE

The village of Gwata is in the province of Manicaland. It is located in an area that used to receive a lot of rainfall, and the weather patterns have generally been conducive for crop production. Due to climate change, rainfall has decreased drastically, resulting in a smaller harvest. This has left a significant portion of the population in a food crisis due to the compounding effects of droughts (Chingarande et al. 2020). Pandemics and the economic situation that have been generally affecting the whole country have not spared Gwata. This area is in a province that was once known as the breadbasket of the country that produced Indigenous crops such as finger millet (*rapoko*), sorghum (*mapfunde*), (*mhunga madhumbe*), tsenza, and brown rice (*chemugomo*), manhangata, and matikiti pumpkins, in addition to maize. The crops grown in Gwata were diverse and nutritious (Page and Page 1991, 4). Hungwe, Masaka, Makuvaro, and Tombo (2020) report that maize has been promoted in preference to other cereal crops like sorghum for the past thirty years. However, the production of maize in Gwata village and countrywide has struggled due to the challenges previously mentioned.

THEORETICAL FRAMEWORK

This study draws on Ellen Messer's concept of food war theory. According to Messer, food wars represent the use of food scarcity for political leverage. A weapon is used to gain an advantage or to defend oneself. Unlike guns and grenades, food does not cause direct physical damage. The effect of using food as a weapon to damage or as an advantage is less apparent, especially if it used in the form of food aid. The aim in using food as a weapon is to weaken the opponent until he or she submits (Messer 1998). In a context where access to food is already limited, it becomes easy to leverage food as a weapon to use in a conflict. The main pathways to achieve this aim are through decreased agricultural production, disruption of markets, and diversion of food aid (Messer 1998; Ekström 2020, 7). The United Nations' Food and Agriculture Organization defines food security as situations in which people have no physical and economic access to sufficient, nutritious, safe food (FAO 2006). In such circumstances, those who have control over the available food can use that privilege to their own advantage or use it to defend themselves. In Gwata village, those who have access to food are using it to propagate their agendas. Generally speaking, the ruling party is using its control over food aid programs to make villagers submit to its demands.

METHODOLOGY

The author conducted a qualitative study involving forty-five participants. Thirty of them were interviewed: fifteen women and fifteen men. A semi-structured interview guide was used that allowed the researcher to develop follow-up questions. The questions mainly focused on ascertaining whether the villagers were accessing enough food and how the distribution of food was being conducted in the area. A focus discussion with fifteen youths (seven female and eight male) was also conducted. The data was thematically analyzed. The data was transcribed and translated into English, which involved reading through the responses and making initial notes. After becoming familiarized with the responses, I coded the data by highlighting phrases and sentences, followed by developing a generation of themes from the codes. Patterns among the codes identified as themes were generated. Throughout the study, confidentiality and anonymity were maintained: informed consent was sought before the onset of the study and pseudonyms were used to protect the participants' identities.

FINDINGS

Some key themes emerged out of my analysis of the interviews. They include farming inputs, the government's and NGOs' emphasis on maize production, denigration of Indigenous farming methods, quantity of welfare benefits distributed by the government, and the solicitation of votes.

Farming inputs

Both the government and NGOs have given the people of Gwata maize seed and fertilizers, which interviewees report do not yield significant harvests. One of the men, *MG1*, said: "All those who used the maize seed which was distributed by the welfare department did not produce much. I used the Indigenous seed (samanyika) which was not from the breeding companies from my previous harvest. My crop was a lot better as compared to that of the seed received from the government." Supporting this, one of the elderly women, *WG4*, added: "The fertilizers are poor quality. There is no change at all in terms of the quality and growth of the crop after applying the fertilizers. This has affected crop production and amount of the harvest. We did not harvest much at all, which means we are faced with a problem of having less sufficient food the greater part of the year."

Commenting on the type of maize seed the government gives to the villagers as part of the inputs, another woman said: "These colored seeds from the government are not effective at all. Our yields are deteriorating a lot. I am not sure if the breeding process is being done properly." Another man also added: "The fertilizers are not helping either. I went to the offices of the organization that gave us the fertilizers to seek clarification why the fertilizers are not causing any growth on the crops. They could not explain. Those who provide the fertilizer cannot even explain why their fertilizers are not effective." The continued distribution of poor-quality fertilizers by the government that do not promote growth of crops and eventually reduce yields is an intentional way of making the rural folk dependent on food aid. As long as they continue to give poor quality fertilizer, the villagers will continue to produce very little food. Therefore, control of farming inputs is a way of controlling food production resulting in villagers being in continual need of food aid. This gives the government hegemonic powers to use food as a weapon.

Emphasis on Maize

The denigration of traditional foods and promotion of maize makes people dependent on this non-Indigenous crop. A youth focus group told the researcher that both the NGOs and the government place greater emphasis on planting maize over other grains. While this practice benefits the NGO, it fails to consider the needs of the villagers. One young person explained: "Rapoko is easy to store. Weevils cannot attack rapoko but maize is vulnerable to weevils and yet they promote the production of maize. Most of the government officials are the owners of the companies that produce and sell maize seed. The reason why they are promoting and preferring the production of maize is for them to have a market for the maize seed they are breeding." An elderly man, *MG2*, had this to say about putting more emphasis on growing maize: "Maize seems now to be the only thing to grow these days. We have the small grain crops that we used to grow, but they are not even mentioned at all. Where is the sorghum, millet, and finger millet we used to grow? These are more nutritious but they do not want us to grow those. It is just a political gimmick."

Another woman, *MG10*, added how food is being weaponized by promoting the growing of maize: "Most seed companies are empires of America. The companies have roots in America. They are doing business. They want to make money. Africa is their business empire. Some seed companies were given licenses to produce seed for our local Indigenous crops, but they are not doing that. Instead, they produce maize seed. The local companies are pushing the agenda of the Americans for them to make money. The Indigenous seeds will not make them make money because everyone is brainwashed to think that maize is the best crop to grow." Expressing her frustration concerning the same issue, another female participant, *WG6*, said: "Besides maize we need other foodstuffs. This noise about growing maize as if we cannot survive without maize surprises me. Our Indigenous vegetables were nutritious. They have medicinal properties to deal with sugar levels, our blood pressure levels. The nongovernmental organizations are saying those vegetables are weeds and not food." Another man, *MG9*, followed with: "The villagers have been colonized even in terms of their diet. Maize is said to be the only food. We had a variety of crops that we were growing. For example, cow peas (Nyemba) do not need a lot of rainfall. In two months, it will be ready to for harvest and it is way more nutritious than maize."

The focus on maize has undermined Indigenous farming practices and has resulted in reduced food production. This lack of production coupled with related impacts on manufacturing has meant that the country remained open to imports, which are usually more expensive than locally produced food, thus increasing the cost of living.

Denigration of Traditional Foods and Farming Techniques

The government compels villagers to grow maize at the expense of other crops that were traditionally grown in the area. One of the elderly women said: "The government is only helping us with the growing of maize and encouraging us to use farming techniques only meant for the production of maize. In this area we used to grow zviyo (rapoko) beans and tsenza, and this will help us have diversity in our diet. Even if there is a drought you will at least harvest something from the drought resistant crops, which would sustain us from one season to another. But these days we are now limited to growing of maize through these government programs."

One of the male participants, *MG10*, also praised Indigenous farming methods, saying: "We used to give our land some rest from time to time. These days shifting cultivation is no longer practiced at all. As a result, the soils are overworked and do not have enough nutrients to help plants grow for one to harvest high yields. We have been practicing the basin farming technique over and over but it has not produced any good results. We only practice it for us to receive the fertilizers and the maize seed. Otherwise, we would have stopped to use it a long time ago." In short, interviewees attested to the ways in which nongovernmental organizations fail to consider Indigenous knowledge when promoting certain approaches to agriculture.

Quantity of Rations

Many people spend a significant amount of time waiting for either NGOs or the state welfare department to bring and distribute food. However, interviewees stated that the quantities the villagers receive are quite small. One of the female participants, *WG15*, complained about the quantities of food provided, saying: "The amount of food handouts for people whom they are not sure of their political affiliation is very little. You spent the whole day waiting only to be given a cup of rice, a bucket of maize, and a gallon of beans. This is not enough to sustain even a small family for a month. But for the ZANU-PF supporters, they get extra portions of whatever is being distributed through the back door."

Participants in the youth discussion group echoed similar sentiments, as they complained that: "The government through the ZANU-PF representatives in the village has been trying to control even food aid from the nongovernmental organizations. At first the staff from the NGOs succumbed to the pressure from the ZANU-PF supporters to distribute the food according to political affiliation such that most opposition supporters did not receive the food rations from NGOs. These days it has improved a bit, even though the amount is also very little. Four families share a fifty-kilogram bag of mealie meal and a two-liter bottle of cooking oil."

Selective Distribution of Food

According to interviewees, food that is meant to be distributed to everyone in the village is now being given to the supporters of the ruling party. The villagers are being forced to become members of the ruling party if they want to receive food from the welfare department. Food is now a tool for obtaining votes. One of the male participants, *MG11*, had this to say: "You are forced to support ZANU-PF if you are to receive the food aid. All supporters of the MDC are not getting any help from the government. If you do not have food in the home, you just have to comply and support the ruling party. The ruling party is demanding that if one is to get food they have to attend ZANU-PF meetings, and to declare publicly their support for the party and to be card holders." One of the female participants, *WG13*, explained how many villagers have become ZANU-PF supporters: "Poverty and hunger forced many to join the ruling party. It was not really by choice. So many of the villagers are now card holders of the ruling party for them to get an allocation of food and the fertilizers. The slogan of ZANU-PF representatives in the area is that 'to receive food 'be a supporter of the ruling party or else you die of hunger."

One of the grandmothers, *WG12*, who also participated in the interviews and supports the opposition party said: "People like us who are staunch supporters of the triple C know we will not get any food aid either from social welfare or the NGOS. They do not declare it publicly why we are not getting the food supply. Some very reliable sources have told us that we are not getting the food because we are Triple C supporters even though we are the rightful beneficiaries of the allocations because we are in the category of the old age who are supposed to get this assistance."

DISCUSSION

The food war theory states that when food is used as a weapon, production is reduced (Messer 1998). The reduction is meant to create high demand and a high deficit amongst people. As evidenced in the interviews I conducted, the government of Zimbabwe has reduced the production of food.

The government has reduced production by diminishing Indigenous crops like rapoko, mhunga, and mapfunde. If other crops were also being grown, food would be available even if maize production was reduced. Besides reducing food production, food crops such as rapoko carry cultural significance among the Shona people of Zimbabwe, to which the Gwata villagers belong. Therefore, by emphasizing the growing of maize instead of Indigenous crops that hold cultural significance, the government is eroding the villagers' culture. Although culture requires protection, the government of Zimbabwe is participating in its destruction. As On (2012) aptly stated, some foods count as "cultural property." Hence, an attack on the food of a people is a calculated act of violence upon the people. The ability to produce their own food in the form of the other Indigenous cereals that are drought resistant would reduce people's dependency on the government for food. Because the government has used food distribution to compel people to support the ruling party, the diversification of food sources might also reduce this dependency and in turn increase political freedom, allowing people to support a political party of their own choice (On 2012, 60).

The government is also reducing production by forcing the villagers to practice the basin farming technique, which has proven not to be effective for some time now in the area. This is when a shallow pit about 30 centimeters long, 15 centimeters wide, and 15–20 centimeters deep is dug in the field and seeds and farming inputs like fertilizer are strategically positioned in the pits (Rusinamhodzi 2015). This technique may be effective in other areas, but according to the interviewees, in Gwata village it has proven not to be effective at all. According to Rusinamhodzi (2015), though this method has been deemed essential to bring to an end the widespread land degradation and to address the incessant food insecurity in the country, it does not necessarily work for all farmers due to differences in resources and locally prevailing biophysical barriers. However, the government is forcing the villagers in Gwata to practice the basin farming technique by making it a condition to receive farming inputs, despite the fact that it has not been producing any positive results. This may be because they want the villagers to continually depend on the government for food. So long as the villagers are harvesting little from their fields, the government is able to maintain control and use food aid as a weapon to make the villagers submit to it. As Maddock (2022) aptly stated, food is now one of the fundamental negotiating tools for most governments.

Furthermore, the food war theory states that if food is used as a weapon there is diversion of food aid as a way of rewarding or punishing certain people. In Gwata village, food aid is being diverted in the sense that food that was meant to be given the elderly people is given to the ruling party supporters simply because its intended recipients are supporters of the opposition party. The food is going to unintended beneficiaries. The elderly villagers who are not getting the allocation they were supposed to get are being punished for being supporters of the opposition party whilst the ruling party supporters are being awarded by getting a bigger portion for supporting the party. By diverting the food from the intended beneficiaries, the government is controlling access and using food as a weapon.

The intention of the government to punish and to bring the villagers who are opposition supporters to submission has been successful, as most of the villagers, as one the participants highlighted, are now card holders. As Messer (1998) has written, the diversion has had the objective to both starve the opponent and to fund and support one's own operation. The ruling party's campaign objective of having more supporters is being funded by the diversion of food aid.

CONCLUSION

In conclusion, in Gwata village, the ruling party is weaponizing food in order to make the villagers submit to its demands. The ruling party is weaponizing food by diverting the food aid. The food aid is not being received by the intended beneficiaries. Furthermore, the government has reduced production especially of maize by not giving everyone inputs and also giving the villagers poor quality fertilizers. This has made food scarce and more expensive, which has in turn made villagers more dependent on food aid, which is largely controlled by the ruling party. Moreover, production of food has been reduced by giving more preference to maize than other crops such finger millet that are more drought resistant. All this has made the villagers dependent on food aid from the government, which has monopolized the distribution of food in the area. For the villagers to survive and not die of hunger, since food prices are generally high and they cannot afford to buy, the villagers have been brought to submission to the demands of the ruling party such as becoming members of the party and attending party meetings. In the end, the ruling party has developed a campaign strategy that relies on using food as a weapon.

SECTION IV

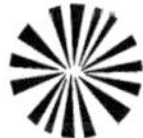

SOUTH ASIAN SUBCONTINENT

10

Taste the Feeling

On "Colanialism" and Its Consequences

Sonakshi Srivastava

THIS CHAPTER EXPLORES the introduction of Coca-Cola to India and its association with modernity, capitalism, ecocolonialism, consumerism, and environmental risks. The "Coca-Colaization" of India was a watershed moment that introduced a "Western" work and lifestyle ethics and aesthetics in Indian households, paving the way for a mimicry that continues to haunt the psyche of Indian culture. All of this, and so much more, has been influenced by a single beverage—Coca-Cola.

Food and drinks are not neutral. Coca-Cola has origins in a first-world country, but influences and continues to influence the lifestyle, environment, and ideas of modernity in third-world countries. In Indian English literature, film, and media, Coca-Cola has been represented as a symbol of modernity, generational divide, Western colonialism, and environmental destruction. This chapter first explores these topics through an analysis of Upamanyu Chatterjee's novel, *English, August* and the Bollywood film *Taal*. It then offers a brief history of Coca-Cola in India. In the final sections, it analyzes the representation of the devastating environmental impact that Coca-Cola production could have in two novels from the 1990s. These novels, I argue, presciently anticipate the environmental problems caused by two Coca-Cola factories in India in the 2000s. Thus, literary representations of Coca-Cola in Indian English literature have not only documented the symbolic history of the drink in India, but have also anticipated the actual effects of its production on the subcontinent.

COCA-COLA IN ENGLISH, *AUGUST* AND *TAAL*

> He sang us a bit of a thumri, excellent, I thought.
>
> "You're interested in music, beyond the noise of Western rock? I'm surprised, I thought you'd be part of our Cola generation."
>
> "My father calls it the generation that doesn't oil its hair."
>
> "That's a nice phrase." Sathe struggled upright to scout for pencil and paper. "I'm stealing it. I've used the Cola generation at least ten times" (Chatterjee 2018, 61).

> A menial with haunted eyes entered, carrying a tray of Campa Cola and nimboo-pani. Agastya wanted both but restrained himself to the latter. The daughter hit the servant in the stomach and screamed, "I want rose sherbet" (Chatterjee 2018, 69).

The aforementioned quotes from Upamanyu Chatterjee's novel, *English, August* reference the key ideas that have defined the consumption of Coca-Cola in India. Viewed by many as being synonymous with "modern," the drink encapsulated the lag between traditional and emerging ways of life—of the generation gap and the associated values (Cola generation vs. the generation that oils its hair, a conflict that pronounces the changing sociocultural conflict), and the "cold (drinks) wars" among all the coolers that proliferated in India after its independence.

In essence, the mention of the drink in the novel warrants some attention despite it being referenced only twice. Published in 1988, the novel embodies the quintessential postcolonial Indian psyche. Agastya Sen, the protagonist of *English, August*, is a hybrid. Born to a Goanese mother and a Bengali father and educated in Anglo-Indian institutes at Darjeeling with a degree from abroad, he finds himself at a startingly disorienting and alienating place after getting assigned to Madna, a dot in the Indian hinterland. A civil servant in training, Agastya's sense of self is uprooted, quite literally and figuratively since he is displaced from the comfort of his hometown in Calcutta as well as his uncle Pultukaku's home in Delhi. His mixed upbringing further fuels discontent. He is described as embodying "a sad mongrel hybridity" with no sense of "coherence" (Chatterjee 2018, 307), so much so that he begins to mimic the Anglo-Indian boys while at school (6) and the Americans as he grows up.

Agastya's condition is symptomatic of the condition of the postcolonial subjects. A sense of fragmentation dictates the postcolonial existence, oscillating between the hatred for the colonizers while at the same time a longing to mimic them as vouched for by Leela Gandhi, who writes, "the desire of the colonizer for the colony is transparent enough but how much more difficult it is to account for the inverse longing of the colonized. Could the colonized deny himself so cruelly? How could he hate the colonizers and yet admire them so passionately?" (Kumar 2010, 41). Agastya's mimicry of the colonizers and Americans earns him the rebuke of his Pultukaku and provides the context for the mention of Coca-Cola in the book.

The generational conflict is evident when Pultukaku is dismayed to discover that Agastya smokes weed, and this dismay is verbalized in a vocabulary that is strongly suggestive of the schism etched by the tug of modernity: "the greatest praise you mimics long for is to be called European junkies. And who is August? In my presence, call him Ogu" (Chatterjee 2018, 36). Agastya and his friends are misfits precisely because they do not fit within the ideas and expectations of their preceding generation. This feeling of displacement is also fueled by the "Americanization" or the neoliberal and neocolonial project made possible by globalization, where the boundaries of the world seem to have contracted by expanding contact. It is no surprise that in the face of the American colonization of India, Agastya dismisses his Pultukaku calling him a mimic and instead labels himself and his generation "the Cola Generation" (61).

While the novel sets the tone for the generational conflict that is embodied by a few sparse invocations of the drink, the conflict finds its culmination in the Bollywood movie *Taal* (Rhythm). Released in 1999, *Taal* was the first significant Bollywood movie to be counted in the top of

Variety's box office list, and it had the advantage of premiering at the Chicago International Film Festival. The premise of the movie is a love story gone awry amidst the conflict between old and modern values. Aishwarya Rai plays the role of the daughter, Mansi, of a spiritual singer who has lost his charm due to the encroachment of modern music technologies. Mansi falls in love with a businessman's son, Manav, played by Akshaye Khanna, and the clash of class distinctions along with the views of the families results in the separation of the lovers. Mansi goes on to become a singing sensation after a music producer strikes a deal with her. The novelty that allows Mansi to gain this newly found popularity is a rendition of her father's spiritual songs. She retouches them with the aid of the modern tools of music production and attains stardom, eventually getting a deal with MTV. Towards the end of the movie, conflicts are resolved, the tense relation between the orthodox, traditional father (Mansi's) and the modern, liberal father of Manav eases, resulting in the reunion of the two lovers.

The premise of the movie makes visible the malady that assailed the Indian psyche, establishing continuity with what was verbalized in Chatterjee's novel—the intergenerational conflict made material with the presence of Coca-Cola. At the juncture of the intergenerational conflict is the question of what is "Indian," and what is "Western/Foreign," how much Indian is Indian, and how much Western is Western? In the movie, Coca-Cola is supposed to heal this unhealed division. In the song "Ishq Bina" (Without Love), coy lovers Mansi and Manav express their love for each other by sharing a bottle of Coca-Cola. While this may not seem strange to the sensibility of non-Indian viewers, it was a rather unique expression of love for Indian viewers because it at once blended the indigenous and foreign notions of expressing love.

Embedded in gastronomic nomenclature, a few excerpts from the lyrics of the song are included below:

> *"ishq bina kya jeena yaaron*
> *Ishq bina kya marna yaaron*
> *Gud se meetha ishq ishq*
> *Imli se khatta ishq ishq."*

This roughly translates as: "what is there to live for if not for love, what is there to die for if not for love. Love, it is sweeter than jaggery, love, it is tangier than tamarind." The lovers exchange forsaken glimpses through curtains, and, in a seemingly complex transaction of love-struck gestures, finally "consume" their love for each other by sipping from the same bottle of Coke.

In the consecutive sequence, the lovers are separated, and it is only towards the end, when the character of Mansi is getting ready to sing a "remix" version of her father's spiritual song—the same "Ishq Bina" that she had previously sung but against an Indian instrumental—that she remembers her long lost love. This remembrance is made material through the presence of a Cola bottle in her hand. The bottle of Coca-Cola offers a remix, a fusion of the two clashing cultures in the movie. The conspicuous role that Coca-Cola plays in the movie can be interpreted as a uniquely cosmopolitan product that attempts to bridge the intergenerational gap in the movie as well as navigate through various lexicons of love, thereby bringing together the "Cola Generation" and the "Generation that oils its hair" (Chatterjee 2018, 61). One might ask if Coca-Cola is necessary to understand such changes. I think that a possible answer might be its fixed formula.

In the Indian foodscape, sherbet, neembu-pani (lemonade), and a host of other Indian coolers are prepared by "andaaz"—a guess work. There is no fixed formula to prepare these coolers. It comes naturally, and also may not, resulting in the drinks being either too sweet, too sour, or too cold—in short, always somehow insufficient. But Coca-Cola, with its fixed formula, its same taste packaged in all bottles, means a shared sip will trigger similar associative memories. It is this sipping that finds a place in the movie. Coca-Cola subverts the prudent Indian diction of love through the replacement of the straw. In *Taal*, drinking from the same bottle without a straw symbolized the lips of the lovers uniting as well as the more general transition towards a "liberal" attitude of embracing love. With its portrayal on the big screen, the message reached a larger audience.

The appearances of the bottle of Coca-Cola within the movie, and particularly within the song "Ishq Bina," afforded a syncretic symbol of the union of India and the West, a perfect drink for a nation that is at once modern and traditional. It sat well with the symbolism of the movie—the rhythm of change and its acceptance through striking a balance. A question then arises: why is Coca-Cola at the interstices of the generational conflict within the movie? Why is the drink's ubiquitous presence a launchpad for the debate between modernity and traditionalism? The answer may be found in the soft drink's checkered past.

A BRIEF HISTORY OF COCA-COLA IN INDIA

Coca-Cola came to India in the year 1950; that is, within three years of its independence from the British rule. The year is significant because it was the year when India declared itself a republic. The company established its bottling plant in Delhi and began full-fledged operations in 1956. Since India had newly gained independence, economic policies were still being formulated. With Jawaharlal Nehru at the helm of national affairs as the prime minister, the political clime was marked by moderate socialist economic reforms. With no definite foreign exchange laws in place, Coca-Cola as a company managed to churn out huge profits. Another soft drink giant, Pepsi, entered the scene but quickly made its exit due to Coca-Cola's gastronomical stronghold over the Indian population. Coca-Cola as a drink had gained so much prominence that its oft-quoted statistic was, "while only 10% of India's villages had safe drinking water, 90% had access to Coca-Cola,"[1] which may be read as an ironic symbol of both indigenous poverty as well as the excess of the influence of a new "West" in post-independence India. The Americanization of India was soon becoming a reality.

However, this reality came to a temporary halt when Nehru's daughter, Indira Gandhi, became India's prime minister. Years of aggression with Pakistan and China along with conflicts with some first-world countries caused Indira Gandhi to enact the Foreign Exchange Act in 1973. The Act required "many multinationals to hand over 60% of the equity in their local subsidiaries to Indian partners."[2] Moreover, to promote local homegrown industries, Gandhi asked the foreign conglomerate to reveal their

---

1. Jeremy Dyck, "How Coca Cola Lost India (And How They Won Her Back)," *BC Digest*, October 10, 2019.

2. Kylie Obermeier, "When India Kicked Out Coca-Cola, Local Sodas Thrived," *GastroObscura*, February 15, 2019.

secret recipe and manufacture their drink locally rather than import it from the United States, thereby driving the final nails in the coffin of the company's exit.

It was only in 1977, though, when the Moraji Desai-led government took national power from Gandhi's regime, that Coca-Cola made its temporary departure from the Indian "cold drinkscape." The company's oft-quoted statistic was also upturned by George Fernandez, the industry minister of that regime, who stated, "when I chucked out Coca-Cola in 1977, I made the point that 90% of India's villages did not have safe drinking water whereas Coke had reached every village. Do we really need Coke? Do we need Pepsi?"[3] Coca-Cola's exit provided a steady foundation for local cold drinks to flourish. To mark the exit of the company, a government sponsored drink was launched in the market—"77", or "double seven." It also served to mark the end of the Emergency and the rise of the Janata Party that formed the government. However, the drink met a fate similar to the Janata Party and fell out of favor within two years. It had failed to charm the taste buds of the Indians because, as the popular idiom goes, "what else can be expected from a government-sponsored drink? It tastes like the government."

The years between 1977 and 1993 saw a host of local drinks flourish. Campa Cola became a household name in lieu of Coca-Cola. However, Campa Cola too fizzled out after the 1989 economic reforms in India, which inaugurated the reentry of Pepsi and Coca-Cola in India. In a feature for the *New York Times* titled "A Revolution Transforms India: Socialism's Out, Free Market In," Edward A. Gargan detailed the events that led to the return of Coca-Cola. The fall of the Soviet Union, India's primary benefactor, and the failing Indian economy propelled prime minister P. V. Narasimha Rao and finance minister Manmohan Singh to formulate the "Eighth Plan" or the "Rao-Manmohan Plan" to revive the ailing industries of India. The plan allowed for the modernization of industries and was characterized by economic liberalization. While it is true that Pepsi came to India before Coca-Cola after it had made its temporary exit, Coca-

3. Edward A. Gargan, "A Revolution Transforms India: Socialism's Out, Free Market In," *New York Times*, March 29, 1992.

Cola was spared from "Indianizing" its name. Unlike Pepsi, which had to prefix "Leher" (Wave) to its name, the belated entry of Coca-Cola allowed it to escape this necessity. At the heart of this Indianization of foreign brand-names is a general mistrust of "cola-nization," as echoed in a 1994 report from *The Los Angeles Times*. The report conveys the strong sense of animosity felt by Indian socialists towards the cold drinks of the West:

> More than half a century ago, with the Japanese army advancing toward the Indian frontier and seemingly unstoppable, Mohandas K. Gandhi, the "Great Soul," launched the call for the British to leave his country, immediately and unconditionally. His target was the injustice and humiliation of colonialism. Now a coalition of alarmed Indian socialists has dusted off his slogan and his tactics of nonviolent protest to battle a more recent foreign foe: "cola-onal-ism," the fizzy, ubiquitous drinks made by Coca-Cola and Pepsi.[4]

When Coca-Cola re-entered India in 1993, it came with the promise of "disintegrating borders" and globalization, which brought about a twofold process of "the particularisation of the universal and the universalisation of the particular" (Robertson 1992, 178). It was this dynamic two-fold process afforded by Coca-Cola that was embedded within the Bollywood movie *Taal* through the presence of the Coke bottle. While a larger point about how and why Coke embodies the "modern" spirit of India has been made by referencing Chatterjee's *English, August*, and *Taal*, it is also important to analyze how Coca-Cola not only influenced India's affects but also its environmental landscape.

COCA-COLA AND THE ENVIRONMENT IN KIRAN DESAI'S *HULLABALLOO IN THE GUAVA ORCHARD* AND ROHINTON MISTRY'S *A FINE BALANCE*

Fernandez's rhetorical reversal of the company's own advertising statistic to describe Coca-Cola's exit from India anticipated a crisis that would come to haunt the future of Coca-Cola upon its eventual return to India—the problem of potable drinking water in places where the company had

4. John-Thor Dahlburg, "Market Focus: Cola's Invasion Stirs Up India's Nationalist Feelings," *Los Angeles Times*, February 15, 1994.

set up its plants. A reference to the potable water scarcity prompted by the construction of Coca-Cola plants can be found in Kiran Desai's novel, *Hullaballoo in the Guava Orchard*. Winner of the Betty Trask Award in 1998, the novel amalgamates themes of desire, hunger, leisure, and work ethics through its protagonist, Sampath. The action of the novel takes place in a household setting and eventually shifts to a guava orchard after Sampath decides that he cannot keep up with the ambitions of his father in particular and of the world in general.

Like Chatterjee's novel, Desai references Coca-Cola only once. However, the scant reference is laden with political and ecological meanings. It is worth noting that both novels are embedded within the matrix of the Indian Administrative Services, a colonial remnant of the Indian Civil Services. In Chatterjee's novel, Agastya is an Indian Administrative Officer who is receives a post in Madna, while in Desai's novel, frequent references to both services and its officers serve to pronounce that colonialism necessarily entails capitalism and as such disallows leisure to its subjects. In an analysis of the novel, Sonakshi Srivastava makes the connection between Coca-Cola, capitalism, and leisure evident by exploring how Sampath and Coca-Cola are "two faces of the same coin—encroaching capitalism" (2022, 8).

The connection between capitalism, leisure, and Coca-Cola is underscored by Fehskens's analysis of the Cola reference and Sampath's introduction to the world through the newspaper clipping. Fehskens writes,

> Desai contextualizes subtly Sampath's flight to the orchard as contemporaneous with Coca-Cola's return to India in 1993. The beverage giant's presence in India was marketed as part of the country's move towards economic liberalization. Since then, environmental activists have drawn repeated attention to the extreme draining of water resources by Coke's bottling plants located in rural and semi-urban regions in the country. Like Kulfi and then like Sampath, Coca-Cola symbolizes a new beginning for the village—rains and a guru—and like the multinational corporation, they also draw all local resources into themselves thus impoverishing the areas around them. The orchard space signifies allegorically

> the inevitable resource crisis imposed on nations in the global south by multinationals (2013, 3).

Moreover, the "rumour" of Coca-Cola's arrival can also be read in tandem with the impending disasters that its arrival would eventually result in—"the news of a scarcity of ground nuts" and "an epidemic of tree frogs" (Desai 1998, 67). The description of the impending doom also evokes a popular Coca-Cola advertisement starring Bollywood actor, Aamir Khan. In this particular advertisement, Khan takes on the role of a farmer and caters to a group of thirsty city girls (who cannot bear the village heat, thereby also contrasting the city to the village) by drawing up a bucket of chilled Coca-Cola bottles from a well. Aamir Khan is heard saying "Thanda matlab Coca-Cola" (A cold beverage means Coca-Cola), thereby implying that Coca-Cola is widely consumed in villages and is no longer just an urban drink, that the reach of Coca-Cola is such that regular Indian coolers have no chance against it, and, consequently, that Coca-Cola is no longer just Coca-Cola but synonymous with any cool/cold drink. Also worth noting is that Aamir Khan's act of drawing Coca-Cola from the well not only lends veracity to the company's initial claim that nearly 90 percent of the Indian population drinks Coke but also highlights what it would ultimately be reproached for—depleting water supplies at the cost of producing Coca-Cola.

A similar sentiment of apprehension is echoed in Rohinton Mistry's novel *A Fine Balance*. As in Chatterjee and Desai's works, the reference to Coca-Cola is only brief but loaded with ecological consequences. The novel was published in 1995, three years before Desai's. Set in mid-1970s India, it narrates the lives of four characters as the National Emergency unfurls. Of particular interest to this paper is the character Maneck Kohlah. Kohlah's father runs a shop and manufactures his own beverage, called "Kohlah Cola." However, "the message was unfavourable. Snuggled amid the goods that the loathsome lorries transported up the mountains was a deadly foe: soft drinks, to stock the new shops and hotels" (Mistry 1995, 220). The clash of the giant corporations and the indigenous brands is made evident when Mr. Kohlah is made an offer that he refuses.

> But the giant corporations had targeted the hills, they had Kaycee in their sights. They infiltrated Mr. Kohlah's territory with their

> board-room arrogance and advertising campaigns and cut-throat techniques. Representatives approached him with a proposition: "Pack up your machines, sign over all rights to Kohlah's Cola, and be an agent for our brand. Come grow with us, and prosper" (220).

The offer made to Kohlah is evocative of how Coca-Cola and Pepsi took over domestic soda brands by acquiring them upon their eventual return to the country. Later in the novel, Kohlah's Cola gets displaced by the "brands which had been selling for years in the big cities," and were now beginning to "saturate the town" (220). The displacement of indigenous brands was only one aspect of encroaching modernity. Modernity also crept into daily life, exerting its influence on everyday decisions. When Mr. Kohlah realizes that his drink "never stood a chance," that his "General Store's backbone was broken, and the secret formula's journey down the generations was nearing its end" (221), he develops a definite plan to secure his son Maneck's future. He decides that Maneck will study "refrigeration and air-conditioning" (221), an industry that "would grow with the nation's prosperity" (221), thereby hinting at how Mr. Kohlah, despite his reservations against the giant corporations, takes cognizance of the fact that their dominance is the new norm.

The "modernization" of towns and villages due to the entry of giant corporations also spells doom for the environment. The alienation that results from this process of "modernization" is enough to propel Mr. Kohlah to give up his life. He cannot bear the loss of his family business, and soon enough, the entire town begins to seem alien to him. "Modernization and expansion were foreign ideas" to him (238) and the construction of factories in the hills troubles his existence further. He watches "helplessly" as:

> The sides of the beautiful hills were becoming gashed and scarred . . . the asphalting began, changing the brown rivers into black, completing the transmogrification of his beloved birthplace where his forefathers had lived in paradise (254).

The resulting loss of paradise causes Mr. Kohlah to lose his mind (256), and in a final attempt to hold onto a chimera of past hopes, he loses balance and falls to his death in the lap of his beloved paradise.

THE FIGHT AGAINST COCA-COLA IN PLACHIMADA AND MEHDIGANJ

The fictionalized accounts of the horrors unleashed by the coming of Coca-Cola in the works of Desai and Mistry cannot be studied in isolation, since they bear witness to the atrocities that the multinational corporation unleashed and continues to unleash on the environment and people of India. The textual details anticipate the horrors of the Plachimada struggle of 2002 in Kerala, a southern state of India. The Plachimada struggle was the earliest and perhaps longest fight against Coca-Cola in India. It all began with the construction of the Coca-Cola plant in the Plachimada district in the year 2000. Sprawling across thirty-four acres of land, the plant produced "5.61 lakh litres of beverages a day, drawing 20 lakh litres of groundwater per day from 6 borewells and 2 ponds."[5] This increased pressure on the water supply and the resulting pollution from the plant caused the Perumatty panchayat—the local governing body that had initially given the company permission to continue its operations in Plachimada—to initiate an inspection against the company and its plant. The ensuing struggle between locals and the Coca-Cola company took a legal turn soon after. In 2002, the locals formed an anti-Coca-Cola committee that went by the name "Coca-Cola Virudha Janakeeya Samara Samithy" (Anti-Coca-Cola People's Struggle Committee). Their sustained protest against the multinational corporation attracted environmentalists, watchdogs, and prominent activists to lend their support to the cause. Multiple investigations, both independent and government-aided, were conducted to study whether the water was being polluted. Most studies concluded that the water was indeed unfit for human consumption because it contained significant quantities of cadmium and lead.[6] The plant was finally shut down in 2005 when its license was revoked, and the company was asked to pay forty-seven million dollars as compensation to the inhabitants of Plachimada for polluting and depleting the water resources.

---

5. Gayatri Raghunandan, "A Look at the Legal Issues Plachimada's Struggle for Water Against Coca-Cola Has Brought Up" *The Wire*, August 20, 2017.

6. Raghunandan, "A Look at the Legal Issues."

Like Plachimada, Mehdiganj in the northern state of Uttar Pradesh bore the brutal brunt of housing a Coca-Cola plant. The Mehdiganj Coca-Cola incident has lately been the focus of many academic case studies. The issues faced by the inhabitants of Mehdiganj were similar to those of the inhabitants of Plachimada. The soft drink plant established in 1999 was polluting and depleting the water resources. However, justice made a belated arrival in Mehdiganj. It was only in 2014 that the Pollution Control Board (PCB) ordered that the factory be shuttered and the government refused to approve the company's expansion plans in Mehdiganj (India Resource Centre). The protests against the factory by the locals were also enmeshed in the old struggle between modernization and traditionalism, Western and the Indigenous. In her fieldwork on the Mehdiganj conflict, Georgina Drew mentions the locals' use of slogans against the firm. Coca-Cola was seen as an American evil that needed to be banished from the country of the holy cow (India). Coca-Cola was accused of driving out local drinks like sugarcane juice, coconut water, and lemon water. The catalog of grievances against the American drink bubbled forth—it was accused of poisoning waters and reducing the water levels (2021, 491).

Plachimada and Mehdiganj are two prominent examples of India's struggle against the terrors of Coca-Cola's capitalist imperialism. The two incidents reflect the anxieties that were first anticipated in the texts of Chatterjee, Desai, and Mistry, and in the movie *Taal*. In his paper "Coca-Cola: A Black Sweet Drink from Trinidad," Daniel Miller writes that the black drink embodies the position of a "meta-symbol" or a "meta-commodity" (2005, 55). The concept of meta-symbol denotes that the object is coded in layers of meanings so much that in this particular case, the term Coca-Cola "comes to stand, not just for a particular soft drink, but also for the problematic nature of commodities in general" (55). It is worth noting then that mentions of the commodity itself are absent in the recently released song "Zaalima Coca-Cola" (2021), which occasions thought about the fact that the mere invocation of Coca-Cola in the Indian imagination brings to one mind not only the liberal ideas of public display of intimacy but also the exploitation of the rural landscape and its people.

CONCLUSION

The oft repeated adage that art reflects society might also be expanded to mean that art anticipates the future of society. The intent of this chapter was to highlight how some Indian novels and films not only captured but also anticipated the pulse of the evolving socio-economic, political, environmental, and cultural changes within the country. This "Cola turn" within the texts not only provides a window into the tensions between different intergenerational ideologies, but also suggests that we be more attentive to the environment that we inhabit.

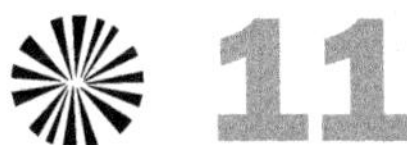 11

The Plight of Dalit Agricultural Workers, Women, and Students in India

Anugrah Brij

IN THE COMPLEX TAPESTRY of India's social fabric, the plight of Dalit agricultural workers, women, and students represents a profound challenge to the nation's ideals of equality, freedom, and justice. Dalits in India continue to face systemic discrimination and oppression in various spheres of life. Within the agricultural sector, where a significant portion of India's workforce is engaged, Dalits often endure exploitative labor conditions, limited access to land ownership, and unequal wages compared to their higher-caste counterparts. Women belonging to the Dalit community face compounded forms of discrimination, subjected not only to caste-based prejudices but also to gender-based violence and sexual and economic exploitation. Moreover, Dalit students encounter barriers to education, stemming from social stigma, lack of resources, and insufficient support systems, hindering their academic advancement and perpetuating cycles of poverty and exclusion. Access to food in India is intertwined with the caste system and entrenched gender inequality.

For many years, policymakers committed to ensuring food security have turned a blind eye to Dalits. Previously known as "untouchables,"

Dalits form the lowest stratum of the castes in India. They face social injustice and atrocities committed by members of the upper castes. This chapter will explore and elucidate caste-based food inequality through the perspectives of Dalit farmers, women, and children. It will detail the history of government actions and laws that have produced and reproduced Dalits' inequal access to food and their position as exploited agricultural laborers. Understanding and addressing these multifaceted challenges is imperative for fostering a more inclusive and equitable society in India.

THE CASTE SYSTEM IN INDIA

The caste system is unique to Indian society. Maintaining it is its dharma, the duty. Over the centuries, it has evolved and has defeated all who challenged it. It remains the backbone of Indian culture and civilization, becoming the source of discrimination against people and the degradation of human personality (Daniel 2019, 4). These are the three reasons why this system, as B. R. Ambedkar (1891–1956) noted, obstructs social peace and justice: graded inequality, fixity of occupation, and fixation of people (Monodeep 2019, 93–148). People are born into their communities, that is, caste. The castes are placed in descending order of purity. So, at the top level are the Brahmin-priests, the second are the Kshatriya-warriors, on the third are the Vaishya-traders, and on the last level are the Shudra-servants. All the rest who are not housed in this graded social order of caste are treated below human dignity and segregated as untouchables.

The word "Dalit" connotes the broken and feeble condition of the so-called untouchables. The term comes from the Sanskrit word "dalita," which means "oppressed" or "broken." The notions of clean and unclean, honor and shame haunt these socially ostracized groups. They are not only perceived as unclean but stand as the most hated beings due to the fixity of occupation described in the Manusmriti. Forced by the circumstances of their birth and poverty, Dalits in India continue to work as sanitation workers: manual scavengers, cleaners of drains, garbage collectors, and sweepers of roads (Bhattacharjee 2019, 3).

Discussions on Dalits in India often revolve around the complex interplay of social, economic, and political factors that have shaped their identity and experiences. Discrimination, segregation, and untouchability are deeply ingrained practices that limit Dalits' access to various aspects of public life. Dalits face systemic exclusion from mainstream society due to their caste-based identity. They are barred from entering temples, using common wells, and participating in many social activities. This exclusion is reinforced by a deeply ingrained social stigma associated with untouchability (Shankar 2007, 254). Though the Indian Constitution abolished untouchability, the oppressed status of Dalits remains a reality. As Zelliot notes, in rural India "they reside in the ostracized quarters, do the dirtiest work, and are not allowed to draw water from the village well which the remaining three castes use . . . In spite of much progress over the last sixty years, Dalits are still at the social and economic bottom of society" (2010, 7).

In rural India, where agriculture remains a cornerstone of the economy and society, Dalit farmers face a unique set of challenges that further exacerbate their already marginalized status. The oppressive caste system, deeply rooted in the fabric of rural life, relegates Dalits to the lowest echelons of society, particularly in agricultural communities. Despite constitutional provisions against untouchability, Dalit farmers are often denied access to productive land, fair wages, and basic amenities crucial for agricultural activities.

The use of food as a weapon to oppress Dalits in India is a deeply rooted and multifaceted issue that reflects the broader social, economic, and cultural inequalities present in India. This practice, which has historical and contemporary dimensions, illustrates how discrimination and social hierarchies manifest themselves in one of the most basic human needs. This chapter delves into the complex ways in which Dalit laborers are subjugated in India's food system, exploring the historical origins, socio-economic implications, and perpetuation of caste-based discrimination. The life quality of the Dalits in India has always been worse than that of the overall Indian population based on factors such as access to health care, life expectancy, education attainability, access to drinking water, and housing (Singh 2009, 535).

DALIT FARMERS

India is a largely rural, agricultural country. The latest census report conducted by the government of India in 2011 suggests that 55 percent of the Indian population engages in agriculture (Kannuri and Jadhav 2021,

563). While a majority of Indian farmers cultivate their own land, Dalit farmers in India continue to work for wages. Thus, instead of calling the Dalit "farmers," the appropriate title for them would be Dalit laborers. According to recent data published by the Census of India, 71 percent of Dalits are landless laborers—they work for wages on land they do not own—and in rural areas, 58.4 percent of Dalit households do not own land at all.[1] This gets grimmer as we look at Dalit-dominated states in India such as Haryana, Punjab, and Bihar, where 85 percent of Dalits are living at the mercy of their landlords.[2] The term "Dalit farmers" refers to a specific segment of India's rural population that intersects two distinct identities—being part of the Dalit community and engaging in agricultural activities. Dalits are systematically excluded from pursuing various occupations and trades considered respectable. This occupational restriction severely limits their economic prospects, forcing them into menial and low-paying jobs. As a result, they face economic exploitation, earning meagre wages for their labor.

Historically, land ownership has been a source of economic power and stability. However, Dalits have largely been denied land ownership and have been relegated to working as agricultural laborers on lands owned by dominant caste groups. This arrangement often leads to exploitative labor practices and further entrenched economic disparities. Agriculture has been the backbone of India's economy for generations, and a significant portion of the population is engaged in farming.[3] Dalit laborers represent a diverse group of individuals who, despite historical disadvantages, contribute to the country's agricultural productivity. From small-scale subsistence farming to labor-intensive activities, Dalit farmers play a pivotal role in rural communities and the nation's food security. About 60 percent of India's

---

1. "The State Should Come to the Rescue of the Landless Dalit Farmer in India," *Hindustan Times*, March 5, 2018.

2. Suraj Yengde, "Landlessness Takes Away Dalits' Legal and Official Validity as Indian Citizens," *Hindustan Times*, July 1, 2019.

3. H. Pathak, J. P. Mishra, and T. Moshapatra, eds., "Indian Agriculture after Independence," Indian agriculture al research, New Delhi, 2022, https://icar.org.in/sites/default/files/2023-02/Indian-Agriculture-after-Independence.pdf.

nearly 1.3 billion people live on less than $3.10 a day, the World Bank's median poverty line. And 21 percent, or more than 250 million people, survive on less than $2 a day.[4] Nearly thirty farmers die each day,[5] driven by debt and distress. Farmer suicides are a significant factor in this equation. A major cause of the farmers' suicides in India has been the increasing burden on the farmers due to inflated prices of agricultural inputs.

The surge in input costs has a significant impact on farmers' financial stability and well-being, and it is often cited as one of the contributing factors to farmers' suicides in many regions. An abrupt increase in input costs, including seeds, fertilizers, pesticides, and machinery, leads to higher production expenses. For small and marginal laborers, who often lack access to credit and financial resources, this creates financial stress and strains their already limited budgets. Be it fertilizers, crop protection chemicals, or even the seeds for cultivation, farming has become more expensive for the already indebted farmers. The input costs, moreover, are not limited to the basic raw materials. Using agricultural equipment and machinery like tractors and submersible pumps adds to already surging costs. Besides, these secondary inputs have themselves become less affordable for small and marginal farmers. If the increased investment in expensive inputs doesn't yield the expected results due to factors like unpredictable weather, pests, or diseases, Dalit laborers face substantial losses. This situation leads to disillusionment and despair, particularly if they have invested heavily or borrowed money to meet these costs. When farmers are unable to cover their increased input costs, they resort to borrowing money from informal lenders or moneylenders at high interest rates. This accumulation of debt, especially in the absence of profitable returns from their produce, create a cycle of indebtedness that becomes increasingly difficult to escape.

The National Crime Records Bureau, an Indian government that collects crime data, pointed out that in 2,474 suicides out of the studied 3,000

4. Moni Basu, "This Is What It Means to Be Poor in India Today," *CNN*, October 13, 2017.

5. Gunisha Kaur, "The Country Where 30 Farmers Die Each Day," *CNN*, March 17, 2022.

farmer suicides in 2015,[6] the victims had unpaid loans from local banks. This is clear enough an indication for drawing correlations between the two. Whether or not the banks had been harassing them, however, is a long-drawn debate and needs more specific empirical evidence. Moreover, a shift away from the usual trend also revealed that only 9.8 percent of farmers' loans came from money lenders.[7] Thus, the pressure or muscle-power of money lenders may be far from being a major driving force, as the Indian government has tended to assert.

Farmer suicides and indebtedness are correlated in many places. While Maharashtra had 1,293 suicides for indebtedness, Karnataka had 946 (Thakur 2018, 19). Both states had one of the highest incidences of farmer suicides as well as indebtedness. The government of India has introduced schemes to mitigate these issues, such as crop insurance and subsidies; however, these measures have failed to address the needs and requirements of the Dalit farmers adequately. The bureaucratic hurdles to accessing these services, coupled with corruption and mismanagement, further exacerbate their challenges. Nearly four hundred thousand farmers died by suicide in India between 1995 and 2018 (Kannunri and Jadhav 2021, 567). The majority of suicides were among people from "backward" castes, including Dalit farmers. The financial and moral debt when accrued within a web of family and caste-related relationships results in patterns of personal and familial humiliation, producing a profound sense of hopelessness. This loss of hope and pervasive humiliation is "cultivated" by a cascade of decisions taken by others with little or no responsibility to the farmers and the land they hope to cultivate as they follow different cultural and financial logic (Kannuri and Jadhav 2021, 567).

These factors create a complex web of economic, emotional, and psychological stressors that can overwhelm farmers, particularly those already facing financial vulnerability. Crop failure leads to immediate and substantial economic losses for farmers. The investments made in seeds, fertilizers, pesticides, labor, and other inputs are lost when the expected yield does

---

6. Deeptiman Tiwary, "In 80% Farmer-Suicides Due to Debt, Loans from Banks, Not Moneylenders," *The Indian Express*, January 7, 2017.

7. Tiwary, "In 80% Farmer-Suicides."

not materialize. For small and marginal farmers who rely heavily on successful harvests for their income, these losses can plunge them deeper into debt and financial instability. The findings should serve as a warning for the worldwide agricultural sector, which is on the frontline of the increasing impacts of climate change. "With their incomes heavily dependent on climate, farmers are on the frontline of this crisis. Climate change is making agriculture an extremely risky, potentially dangerous, and loss-making endeavor for farmers, and it's increasing their risk of suicide."[8]

The Three Farm Laws

Between 2020 and 2024, three controversial farm laws were passed in India: the Farmers' Produce Trade and Commerce (Promotion and Facilitation) Act, the Farmers (Empowerment and Protection) Agreement on Price Assurance and Farm Services Act, and the Essential Commodities (Amendment) Act. The laws have been met with widespread protests and criticism. These laws have disproportionately benefited agribusiness and corporate interests rather than addressing the concerns of small and marginalized farmers.[9] The perception that the three farm laws in India have favored capitalists over farmers stems from concerns over increased corporate influence, potential exploitation, lack of safeguards, and possible impacts on existing support mechanisms like the Minimum Support Price (MSP). Critics contend that the laws fail to address the structural issues that impact small and marginalized farmers, potentially leaving them at the mercy of powerful corporate interests.

First, the Farmers' Produce Trade and Commerce (Promotion and Facilitation) Act, one of the key components of India's recent agricultural reforms, has garnered significant attention and debate. This legislation allows farmers to sell their produce outside the purview of Agricultural Produce Market

8. International Institute for Environment and Development, "Climate Change Driving Increase in Farmer Suicides in India," 2023, https://www.iied.org/climate-change-driving-increase-farmer-suicides-india.

9. "Agricultural Bills Are Anti-farmer, Will Benefit MNCs, says Maniarasan," *The Hindu*, September 21, 2020, https://www.thehindu.com/news/national/tamil-nadu/agriculture-bills-are-anti-farmer-will-benefit-mncs-says-maniarasan/article61704236.ece.

Committees (APMCs) or traditional markets. Proponents of this act argue that it fosters competition in agricultural markets and reduces the role of intermediaries, which could lead to increased income for farmers. However, the farmers are of the view that this deregulation potentially exposes them to the influence of large corporate buyers who may manipulate prices, exploiting the farmers' limited bargaining power. Large corporations, equipped with financial resources, could stockpile commodities, exert control over prices, and leave farmers vulnerable to market fluctuations.[10]

Second is the Farmers (Empowerment and Protection) Agreement on Price Assurance and Farm Services Act, which seeks to facilitate contract farming agreements between farmers and agribusinesses. On the surface, this could provide farmers with access to modern technology and a guaranteed market for their goods. However, concerns arise regarding the potential for corporations to impose unfair contracts, exploiting the information gap between farmers and powerful corporations. This information asymmetry could lead to farmers entering into unfavorable agreements, ultimately resulting in the loss of their land and income.[11]

Third, the Essential Commodities (Amendment) Act has removed specific agricultural commodities such as cereals, pulses, oilseeds, edible oils, onions, and potatoes from the list of essential commodities. This alteration enables traders and corporations to stockpile these commodities without government intervention during price fluctuations. Farmers argue that this could potentially result in artificial scarcity, hoarding, and price manipulation, harming both consumers and small-scale farmers.[12]

One of the overarching concerns related to these agricultural reforms is the potential impact on the Minimum Support Price (MSP) system. While the laws themselves do not directly affect the MSP, farmers worry

---

10. PRS Legislative Research, "The Farmers' Produce Trade and Commerce (Promotion and Facilitation) Bill, 2020," https://prsindia.org/billtrack/the-farmers-produce-trade-and-commerce-promotion-and-facilitation-bill-2020.

11. "Agricultural Reforms: Here's a Look at Key Measures in the Legislation Passed in Lok Sabha—Landmark Agricultural Reforms," *The Economic Times*, September 19, 2020.

12. K. B. Pragati, "Explainer: Why Are the Agriculture Bills Being Opposed," *The Hindu*, November 28, 2021.

that the deregulated markets created by these reforms could undermine the MSP system. Corporations may opt to purchase produce at prices below the MSP, rendering the MSP ineffective and endangering farmers' income security. The core argument against these agricultural reforms centers on the perceived lack of safeguards for farmers, especially small and marginalized ones. Scholars assert that the laws fail to incorporate adequate protective measures to shield farmers from potential exploitation by corporate entities. Small-scale farmers, often constrained by limited legal and financial resources, may struggle to negotiate fair terms with influential corporate buyers, placing them at a disadvantage. Therefore, driven by distress either the farmers resort to measure such as suicides or they turn towards the urban cities in search of employment, thus leaving their families.

Dalit Women in India

"As crops wither and livestock perish, tens of thousands of male community members migrate in search of food, water, and shelter, leaving behind their women, children and older family members who are vulnerable to human traffickers."[13] "Dalit women are among the most oppressed communities in the world," reports the BBC.[14] Dalit women die younger than dominant caste women, and nutrition and health have always been a struggle for them.[15]

In an unregulated market with no safeguards, India's disempowered female farmers have the most to lose. Seventy-one percent of women get their livelihood from farming.[16] These women, most of whom are Dalits, are largely invisible in this sector. Most do not own any land at all, and, if they do, it is small in size. They earn less than male laborers and have virtually no power to negotiate prices of wages. Dalit women experience dis-

---

13. Rina Chandran, "Hunger, Child Marriage, Prostitution—India Drought Hurts Women, Low-Caste Dalits More," *Reuters*, May 23, 2016.

14. Soutik Biswas, "Hathras Case: Dalit Women Are Among the Most Oppressed in the World," *BBC*, October 6, 2020.

15. Ajai Sreevatsan Ashwaq Masoodi, "Dalit Women in India Die Younger than Upper Caste Counterparts: Report," *Mint*, June 6, 2018.

16. Food and Agriculture Organization of the United Nations, "FAO in India: India at a Glance," https://www.fao.org/india/fao-in-india/india-at-a-glance/en/.

crimination at the intersection of their caste and gender identities. They are often relegated to the lowest socioeconomic strata, limiting their access to education, employment, and resources. This lack of access extends to food, as they may be denied proper nutrition, healthcare, and adequate food supplies due to their lower social status. In some cases, dominant caste groups may deliberately withhold food from Dalit women as a means of asserting their dominance and reinforcing traditional hierarchies. Dalit women are disproportionately engaged in agricultural labor, often as landless laborers. They face exploitation in the form of meagre wages, hazardous working conditions, and limited access to nutritious food. Their contribution to food production is vital, yet they themselves may not benefit from it. The restriction to the access of food also perpetuates a sense of social exclusion and humiliation.

Dalit women face dual marginalization. They also experience oppression and dehumanization. Higher levels of food insecurity and hunger lead women to exchange food for sex.[17] In many cases of the devadasi system (women being wives of God in temples), these women are raped by priests who oversee the temple.[18] They commit themselves as devotees, and the Brahminical structure maintains its hegemony by controlling the women. It may be contended that Dalit women should consider pursuing a profession as a means to address their socio-economic challenges, but Dalit women are often prevented from pursuing professions. In a notable instance in India, students declined to consume meals prepared by Dalit women.[19] Alarmingly, even law enforcement agencies have been observed to abstain from intervention in such occurrences, largely due to affiliations with higher caste groups. Consequently, Dalit women endure the contin-

---

17. Sustainable Development, "Ending hunger and achieving food security for all: Answers to guiding questions–UNFPA," https://sustainabledevelopment.un.org/content/documents/26475Answers_to_guiding_questions_UNFPA.pdf.

18. V. Bharathi Harishankar and M. Priyamvadha, "Exploitation of Women as Devadasis and Its Associated Evils," National Commission for Women, New Delhi, https://ncwapps.nic.in/pdfReports/Exploitation_of_Women_as_Devadasis_and_its_Associated_Evils_Report.pdf.

19. Ashish Chauhan, "Gujarat: OBC Kids Refuse Food Made by Dalit." *Times of India*, August 4, 2022.

uing hardships of heightened poverty, gender discrimination, and class-based disparities within the purview of socio-economic deprivations.

This endemic confluence of gender and caste systems underscores a profound imbalance in sociopolitical power dynamics.[20] In rural Indian villages, educational institutions are predominantly attended by children from upper caste backgrounds, while Dalit children often find themselves compelled to engage in income-generating activities to alleviate their family's financial burdens. The midday meal schemes, an initiative primarily designed to ameliorate the nutritional well-being of school-attending children across India, have regrettably become skewed toward favoring upper-caste students. This disproportionate allocation of benefits adversely affects the employment prospects of Dalit women. It is imperative to underscore that the Dalit women often ostracized in this context are actively involved in the cultivation and harvesting of the crops destined for these meals. The influence of the caste system has profoundly infiltrated the minds of young students, leading them to reject food based on notions of purity expounded in their sacred texts. Consequently, this deep-seated discrimination undermines the employment opportunities for Dalit women and systematically obstructs their avenues for social and economic advancement. Such systemic obstacles can be attributed to the intersecting structures of patriarchy and casteism pervasive within Indian society.

Dalit women suffer from the intentional denial of access to food, nutrition, and related resources as a form of discrimination and oppression. This practice reflects the intersection of caste-based discrimination and gender inequality, resulting in a grave violation of human rights. Historically marginalized and oppressed, Dalit women often face compounded challenges, making them particularly vulnerable to such tactics. This practice underscores the urgent need for comprehensive initiatives that challenge discriminatory norms, ensure access to resources, and promote the rights and well-being of Dalit women within the broader framework of social justice and human rights.

20. Insight IAS, "Challenges Faced by Dalit Women," blog, https://www.insightsonindia.com/social-justice/issues-related-to-sc-st/dalit-women/challenges-faced-by-dalit-women/.

Dalit Students

Largely, Dalit infants do not have adequate nourishment, which can cause lifelong developmental disabilities (Daniel 2019, 8). Those who survive are taunted with derogatory remarks due to reservation that is enshrined in the India constitution within the spheres of Indian society.

Developmental disabilities caused by malnutrition in infancy are further exacerbated by malnutrition, which has a cyclical relationship with unemployment. In the educational landscape of India, the pursuit of intellectual freedom is often met with significant challenges, including physical and psychological aggression. A notable example of this phenomenon transpired at the prestigious Indian Institute of Technology (IIT) Madras, a globally recognized university.[21] In this context, a student faced punishment for participating in a "beef fest," which, regrettably, has profound repercussions on the multifaceted development of individuals encompassing their motor, sensory, cognitive, social, and emotional facets.[22] On a social level, he was then ostracized by his fellow students. On a political level, when students endeavor to voice their dissent against the oppressive forces, they frequently encounter ostracization, culminating in deleterious consequences for their mental well-being. On an economic level, the affordability of the food of their choice is impacted, and on the mental level, the marginalization is exacerbated by the fact that a significant portion of the student body hails from upper-caste communities, which accentuates the isolation experienced by those who advocate for change. Consequently, many individuals descend into the abyss of depression, and in the direst of circumstances, reminiscent of the tragic case of Rohit Vemula,[23] they resort to the ultimate act of self-harm, leading to tragic outcomes.

---

21. Education Desk, "Here's How IIT's Performed in QS World University Rankings 2024," *The Indian Express*, July 7, 2023.

22. Express Web Desk, "IIT Madras Student Thrashed by ABVP for Attending 'Beef Fest'," *The Indian Express*, May 30, 2017.

23. Rohith Vemula was a student who died fighting for Dalit rights on a University Campus. For more, see Omer Farooq, "Rohith Vemula: The Student Who Died for Dalit Rights," *BBC*, January 19, 2016.

At a profound societal level, these individuals are confronted with the disheartening reality of isolation, stemming from their caste affiliation and economic circumstances, which effectively render them as outcasts. On a political front, their experiences are marred by both physical and psychological oppression, exacerbated by the lamentable absence of concrete reservation policies tailored to ameliorate their plight. Meanwhile, the economic dimension further compounds their predicament, depriving them of the liberty to partake in the sustenance of their choosing. This multilayered oppression, at its core, leaves a devastating imprint on their emotional well-being, casting a pervasive shadow of depression. In conclusion, this intricate tapestry of challenges, interwoven with social, political, economic, and emotional dimensions, underscores the dire circumstances faced by these marginalized individuals, necessitating concerted efforts to rectify these systemic injustices.

CONCLUSION

The government must address the issues faced by Dalits in India by conducting surveys, feedback sessions, and inquiries. The policy makers, often educated at prestigious institutions like Harvard and Stanford, are far away from the ground realities experienced by Dalit farmers.[24] It is imperative to diversify the composition of decision-making bodies, both at the national and regional levels. This includes government offices, think tanks, and advisory committees. Representation from marginalized communities, including Dalits, should be increased to ensure that policies and solutions are informed by a range of perspectives and experiences. Policymakers should engage directly with Dalit communities and farmers. This means fostering a more immersive and participatory approach, where policymakers spend time understanding the daily challenges and aspirations of Dalits. Field visits, discussions, and interactions at the grassroots level can help policymakers gain a deeper understanding of the issues. Policymakers should be encouraged to initiate reforms and policies that address the unique issues of Dalit farmers. These policies may include land reforms,

24. Vincent Diaz, "Nero's Guests" by P. Sainath, documentary, https://www.youtube.com/watch?v=Wti7W0xANDA.

access to credit, agricultural extension services, and market linkages tailored to the needs of Dalits. Effective implementation and monitoring mechanisms should also be put in place. Civil society organizations, academic institutions, and advocacy groups can play a crucial role in raising public awareness about the challenges faced by Dalit farmers. Advocacy efforts should aim to put pressure on policymakers to prioritize issues related to Dalits and ensure their inclusion in mainstream policy agendas.

The recognition of Dalits as equal human beings, deserving of the same rights and opportunities as others, is an essential element to their liberation. Core human values of love, justice, and compassion underpin this approach to help Dalits break free from the shackles of the caste system and attain a life of freedom and independence. Society must recognize the inherent worth and dignity of every individual. This recognition implies that Dalits, like all people, have a natural right to live free from discrimination and oppression based on their caste. Their liberation begins with acknowledging their full humanity. The liberative approach underscores the importance of love and compassion towards Dalits. We ought to show love and compassion to marginalized and oppressed individuals. This approach encourages all indiviuals to engage with Dalits on a personal and communal level, offering support, empathy, and practical assistance. We ought to place a strong emphasis on justice. From a humanitarian point of view it is crucial to advocate for the rights and equality of Dalits. This includes working towards legal reforms and social changes that eradicate discriminatory practices, ensuring that Dalits have access to education, employment, and other opportunities.

We can educate ourselves and others about the historical injustices faced by Dalits and the ongoing challenges they encounter. By raising awareness about caste-based discrimination and its impact, we can advocate for policy reforms and legislative measures aimed at addressing caste-based discrimination and promoting Dalit rights. This would involve supporting Dalit-led organizations, participating in protests and demonstrations, and lobbying policymakers for change. We can support Dalit-owned businesses and initiatives that promote economic empowerment within Dalit communities. By providing financial assistance, mentorship, and market access, individuals can help Dalit entrepreneurs thrive and break the cycle of poverty.

The plight of Dalit agricultural workers, women, and students in India remains a pressing concern that demands urgent attention and action. Despite constitutional provisions and affirmative action policies, deep-rooted social hierarchies and systemic discrimination continue to marginalize Dalits, perpetuating cycles of poverty, exploitation, and exclusion. B. R. Ambedkar highlighted the enduring struggles faced by Dalits in his writings and speeches. He emphasized the need for social reform, economic empowerment, and educational opportunities to uplift Dalits from centuries of oppression. Ambedkar's vision of a more just and inclusive society underscores the importance of addressing the specific challenges faced by Dalit agricultural workers, women, and students. Dalit scholars and activists have extensively documented the intersecting forms of discrimination experienced by Dalit communities across various spheres of life. From landlessness and exploitation in agriculture to gender-based violence and limited access to education, Dalits confront multifaceted barriers that hinder their socio-economic advancement. In conclusion, the struggle for Dalit rights is inseparable from the broader quest for social justice and equality in India. By amplifying the voices of Dalit scholars and activists, advocating for policy reforms, and promoting grassroots empowerment initiatives, we can work towards a more inclusive and equitable society where every individual, regardless of caste or gender, can fulfill their potential and contribute to the nation's progress.

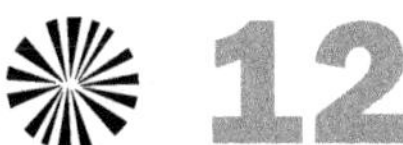

12

Kenzong Rinpoche, Precious Corn
Traditional Snacks in the Making of Interdimensional Nourishment and Food Sovereignty in the Sikkim Himalayas

Kalzang Dorjee Bhutia

In western Sikkim, a cup of tea and offering of snacks is a standard part of any social visit, whether it be for official purposes or to catch up with family members. One of the most famous producers of tea in the world, Darjeeling, is adjacent to Sikkim and was part of the state until it was annexed by British colonial authorities in 1835. The annexation of Darjeeling marked the beginning of British encroachment into the kingdom. By the time Sikkim was annexed by the Republic of India in 1975, political administration, especially for external affairs, had long been controlled by British and then, after 1947, Indian political officers. Tea and sovereignty are therefore entangled in Sikkim, and so are the snacks served with tea. Along with tea, a visitor to a house or office in western Sikkim is often offered mass-produced biscuits made by Indian companies including Parle, or savory items like chips and bhujia produced by Haldiram's or international brands such as PepsiCo. These imported goods represent the importation of new foods and ideas about nourishment into Sikkim.

However, along with these processed salty and sugary snacks, other less widely known snacks are also offered. These include kyabse, ornate plaited snacks made from maida flour; zero, a fried snack that resembles a bird's nest made from rice powder; saiyo, made from dried rice; and byasu chadung, a unique egg-shaped snack made from corn. These snacks are all consumed by the many ethnic and cultural groups in western Sikkim and serve as offerings to guests both human and more-than-human. In western Sikkim, more-than-human guests and co-residents in the land are spirits that people interact with through religious rituals and daily practices across different cosmologies. To Buddhist communities in the region, these spirits are considered to be *chökyong yullha zhidak*, protectors of the land and multidimensional residents of Sikkim. These beings may take on different forms and reside in all elements of the local environment, including in the mountains that tower over western Sikkim, the trees of Sikkim's forests, and the hearth of the kitchens of the households. Food offerings are important events in ritual life and crucial to maintaining interdimensional balance between humans and more-than-human forces.[1] The making of western Sikkimese food, and specifically snacks, involves different elements of the environment, from planting seeds, to harvesting fruits, grains, and vegetables, to making and consuming different snacks. The processes of making as well as eating and sharing are part of what brings together different residents, both seen and unseen, human and non-human, in Sikkim.

What happens then when these processes are disrupted? The arrival of mass-produced snacks and beverages in Sikkim has coincided with the development of colonial infrastructure in the region, as a form of what English literature scholar Craig Santos Perez and anthropologist Sophie Chao has called "gastrocolonialism" (Chao 2022, 811).[2] The health and

1. For more on Sikkimese Buddhist traditions related to the spirits of the land, see Bhutia 2021a; and Bhutia 2022, 175–86.

2. Craig Santos Perez, "Facing Hawai'i's Future," *Kenyon Review*, July 10, 2013, http://kenyonreview.org/2013/07/facing-hawai i s-future-book-review/.

well-being of local human communities have been deeply impacted by the introduction of these new snacks as commodities; however, traditional snack foods continue to be sought out, even if they are less frequently made by individual households. This chapter will illustrate the significance of these traditional snack foodways for local humans and more-than-humans as a form of sovereignty and as an indicator of community well-being. I will focus on corn (also known as maize, zea mays) as a traditional historical crop, because it is a central ingredient for both traditional and newly introduced snack foods. By examining its historical role for western Sikkimese Indigenous communities, I will interrogate how changing patterns of production and consumption impact ways of knowing and relating to the land and food by drawing on historical, textual, and ethnographic research in my community, the Lhopo (also known as Bhutia) people. Other Indigenous communities in Sikkim and around the world also acknowledge the agency and power of corn to nourish relatedness. Corn has been eaten in the highlands of Mexico for more than six thousand years (Garcia-Weyandt 2023, 1) and has since spread globally through processes of trade and empire (Warman 2003, 1). For example, Wixárika families in Mexico honor and care for corn as a relative. Cyndy Garcia-Weyandt writes that "Yuawima ('Blue Corn') was the first Corn maid to be part of the first farmer's family. She was a Corn-person and lived with Watakame ('First farmer') to provide seeds. Watakame cultivated the land as part of the many rituals to maintain kinship with not only Yuawima but also all 'other-than-human' beings including Tatéi Niwetsika ('Our Mother Corn')."[3] Agricultural researchers have recently argued that Sikkim and other northeast Indian states may be "the secondary center of origins of maize" due to the "resemblance" between Sikkimese corn and other "primitive" forms (Borah, et al. 2012, 211). This is affirmed by oral traditions within different Sikkimese communities. Like Wixárika families in Mexico, many communities in Sikkim also hold corn to be an agent in the making of relations across time, space, and dimensions.

3. Cyndy Garcia-Weyandt, "Curing with our Mother Corn," *The Jugaad Project*, October 27, 2021, www.thejugaadproject.pub/mother-corn.

In these cross-cultural settings, thinking about how corn brings sustenance and healing while also forging relations and kinship can help facilitate an understanding of how this important grain, vegetable, and fruit remains central to many cosmologies, even as it is extracted and appropriated by major commercial agro-industrial corporations (Warman 2003, 1–2). These local ways of knowing and eating corn are representative of food sovereignty and can counter extractive approaches to the land by emphasizing reciprocity between humans and more-than-humans (Barbora et al. 2023, 4).

There are many ways to relate to corn in Sikkim. This chapter delves into some of these by examining how they interact with other ways to relate to the land, corn as a specific snack that brings humans and more-than-humans together, and the different ways corn is valued across dimensions. I will draw on narratives from ethnographic research, historical and ritual texts, and agricultural knowledge from my family to illustrate these explorations. In centering these perspectives, this chapter includes critical discussion but emphasizes local ways of knowing as a form of food sovereignty. This focus has been inspired by Lotha Naga anthropologist Dolly Kikon's research, which emphasizes "seemingly ordinary practices and conversations" about food as a way to understand social relations (Kikon 2021, 376).

INTERDIMENSIONAL NOURISHMENT IN SIKKIM: FOOD AS A WAY TO UNDERSTAND RELATIONS WITH THE LAND

Sikkim is a diverse state that is home to many cultural communities and cosmologies,[4] and therefore, many different foodways and cosmologies that connect land and food (Tamang 2001, 107; and Tamang 2005, 1). The first Indigenous people of Sikkim, the Rong (also known as Lepcha, an appellation from the colonial period), trace their genealogy to the snows of Kanchendzonga, the third highest mountain in the world, as the first people were created by the mother creator Itbudebu Rum from snow (Lepcha 2021, 49–50). For as long as oral tradition has persisted, Rong

4. For a helpful introduction to and overview of contemporary Sikkim's diverse cultures and ethnic groups, see Chettri 2015.

communities have cared for their origin mountain through ritual traditions. Some of these rituals involved offering corn before harvesting crops (Borah et al., 2012, 212). When later communities arrived, they joined with the Rong in forms of ritual care that often incorporated crops as ritual offerings and agents. These relationships were complicated and could be marked by conflict, but they have also led to a sharing of cosmovisions and the emergence of localized religious traditions that include multiple layers of cultural knowledge.

Local traditions met with Buddhism early on. In traditional narratives, Buddhism entered Sikkim in the eighth century with the arrival of the popular Inner Asian Buddhist traveler and Tantric teacher, Guru Rinpoche.[5] He visited Sikkim as part of his broader travels throughout Tibet and the Himalayas and named Sikkim the Beyul Demojong, or Hidden Valley of Rice. This name came from widely available wild rice, along with many other edible plants. In the prophetic texts that he left for Buddhists in the landscape, he stated that the land in Beyul Demojong was very fertile. In one of these prophetic texts, he states:

> There are about 155 varieties of fruits with different tastes and nutritional values. [These include] a walnut that tastes like butter; a fruit known as wallay . . . and a grape with the taste of wine. There are fruits called tingding with the taste of meat, and sedey, which can be eaten as the equivalent of an entire meal; turnips, and thirty-seven other types of root vegetables are available. There are twenty different varieties of garlic. Altogether, among the edible plants, there are 360 varieties available. There are wild radishes, along with tsolay, nyolay, grapes in the valley. In the trees, among the rocks and hanging from the cliffs there are beehives (Tshering 2008, translated by the author).

From this classical Tibetan prophetic text, we can see how from a very early period in the Buddhist engagement with Sikkim, foodways were an important manifestation of the auspiciousness and abundance of the

5. For more on the cultural role and different historical traditions associated with Guru Rinpoche, see Hirshberg 2016.

land, its suitability for residence, and an important way people interacted with the land.

Guru Rinpoche's prophecies were part of a wider corpus of stories that explain the migration of the Lhopo community, my ancestors, from eastern Tibet to Sikkim in the thirteenth century CE. Along with the Rong, Limboo, and Mangar communities, our community are considered Indigenous in contemporary state discourse and cultural practice. Apart from the Rong people, who are originally from the region, each of these communities has histories of migration. Part of what makes us Indigenous in this place are long histories of dwelling, and particularly, foodways. Many of our foods were shared with the first Rong communities and other communities through intermarriage and neighborly generosity. Many other communities have come since and shared their foodways, leading to great variety and diversity. This idea of hospitality and generosity is why I often choose to translate Beyul Demojong as the Valley of Abundance, as a way to acknowledge the power and fertility of the land.

Many tales of living together in the land are linked by the fact they are all associated with stories of Guru Rinpoche and his travels. In these stories, he left many seeds to be sown by human residents in the land. However, as demonstrated in the quote from the prophetic text above, there were already many seeds here. The Guru Rinpoche stories therefore give us important insight into the different layers of food histories, allowing us to think about what constitutes a native crop and what is introduced, and how the introduction of certain foods has accompanied other forms of cultural interaction and transformation. The seeds referenced in these stories are still passed through village communities, taken from the first harvest of the year and kept for planting the next year, and also as part of Pang Lhabsol, the annual Buddhist ritual offering to the mighty mountain deity, Kanchendzonga.[6]

The first of the seeds that Guru Rinpoche was held to have left were seeds of paddy, or rice, which is a staple for all of the different ethnic and cultural communities of Sikkim. In the Lhopo language, we call rice dre,

6. For more on this ritual tradition, see Bhutia 2021b.

or bya. In Buddhist oral traditions, it is said that Guru Rinpoche planted his walking stick in Chungthang in northern Sikkim, and that the walking stick became a tree, and from his bowl, he planted one grain of rice, which led rice to grow abundantly in Chungthang. This was one of the many types of rice that grow in Sikkim. The name Beyul Demojong, which is most commonly translated the Hidden Valley of Rice, tells us that rice was already present, as do many Rong oral and ritual traditions, and so Guru Rinpoche's rice was another type of rice species. The Guru Rinpoche story suggests how varied species of rice came to be planted and flourished in Sikkim.

The second of the seeds associated with Guru Rinpoche is millet, or minchak. There is some debate over whether millet was introduced at the time of Guru Rinpoche or whether it was already present, but it is found in many places and used for a variety of foods. It can be roasted and can be turned into flour for bread. Importantly, it is used for making chang—millet beer—which is widely consumed. The process of fermentation has led chang to be positively associated with abundance, which in turn has occasioned its wide use in ritual. Chang has low alcohol by volume and contains microbes that are beneficial for stomach bacteria, which have contributed to its perception as a medicinal drink. This stands in contrast with forms of alcohol that were later introduced from abroad.

The third is corn, or kenzong. Corn is so widely used it[7] is even sometimes called "Kenzong Rinpoche," or precious one. This title is normally reserved for human Buddhist teachers, and its use to refer to corn gestures towards the significance of corn as a staple. Sikkim has a rich variety of types of corn. In western Sikkim, yellow and white corns are most common, and purple corn is also grown. Altitude impacts the planting and growing cycle of corn. At the altitude of my village in western Sikkim, around five thousand feet, corn seeds are sown in February. Corn grows and can begin to be plucked in July but must be boiled or roasted before it is eaten at this time as the corn is particularly hard. In early August,

7. I acknowledge here that referring to corn as "it" can erase a form of relationship. I have used "it" in this chapter for consistency but not as a way to erase the ability for corn to act as an agent.

corn can be plucked to be used to make byasu chadung, corn-based snacks, and in late August the remaining corn is harvested and stored outside of homes in wooden structures known as kenzong tangra. When the corn is hung outside in the tangra, people keep the husk on the corn (which is called kenzong shoka in the Lhopo language). When people eventually eat the corn, the husk is removed and used for weaving baskets and small cushions to sit on outside.

CORN-BASED SNACKS IN SIKKIM: MAKING RELATIONS WITH CORN

These wooden structures are made with great care because corn is an important staple for Lhopo communities in western Sikkim. There are many ways to eat corn: on the cob after it has been boiled until it becomes brilliant yellow, or cooked on the fire until it becomes reddish brown. Fresh hard kenzong is also made into powder and cooked in hot water. When the water becomes dried, the remaining corn powder is eaten with pickles or buttermilk. This preparation is known as drem in the Lhopo language and dero in the Nepali language. Once it gets more mature in the field, it can be used to make many types of dishes or snacks, including being eaten in chunks with dairy products, chutney, or gundruk (a fermented mustard leaf dish eaten throughout the Sikkimese Himalayas and in Nepal). Corn can also be used to make fermented alcohol, especially arak, or clear alcohol, which is enjoyed by humans in social settings and also offered to protector deities in rituals. Corn also gives sustenance to nonhuman animals who live in the land. We grind corn to make powder that can be used to feed humans and cows, pigs, horses, chickens, ducks, geese, and goats. The corn husk is also used in animal feed, especially for cows. On some mornings, farmers find their corn fields flattened with large round prints from bears, who have ventured into the fields for a snack during the night. Birds also frequently eat discarded corn. The abundance of corn for multiple human and nonhuman residents of Sikkim, and its ability to remain edible for long periods of time, is part of why it is called Kenzong Rinpoche, as it provided nourishment in times of scarcity and famine.

Among humans, corn is most famous for its association with snacks, and especially for making byasu chadung. Byasu chadung is another distinctive snack that I have only found in Sikkim, though it is often served with other popular trans-Himalayan snack foods, including kyabse. Byasu chadung is made by soaking corn overnight, then roasting and beating into a cup shape. The beating of the corn into a consistency that will allow it to be molded into the distinctive egg-like shape of byasu chadung is a lengthy process. The soaked corn is drained, and the remaining corn liquid is then put into a stone bowl and beaten with a wooden mallet. Two people lift the mallet together to beat the corn and form cups from the smashed pulp.

This beating is a lengthy and skilled process. When we were children, our parents warned us to remain mindful of the sores and blisters that develop on the hands of people who make the byasu chadung; they told us to pray to ease the suffering of their blisters. Consuming byasu chadung therefore carries with it some of the same ethical responsibility of consuming other types of food connected to sentient beings, including nonhuman animal products such as dairy milk and meat. Before these items are consumed in Sikkimese Buddhist households, some people will pray for the well-being of all sentient beings, directing compassion towards beings who may have suffered in order for their food to make it to the table. This tradition of prayer encourages reciprocity and awareness of where food comes from and how the growth, harvesting, and preparation of food are all contingent on other beings. Growing, harvesting, preparing, and consuming corn are all activities that rely on relationships then—among the corn, different spirits of the soil and land, nonhuman animals and birds that help to carry and fertilize the seeds, and humans.

Knowledge of these relationships is passed on through family lineages as part of agricultural, ritual, and food preparation traditions. This knowledge is especially important, because byasu chadung, along with other traditional snacks, are often made especially in preparation for significant family events, including rituals such as funerals, death memorials, and life strengthening rituals, along with weddings and new house and business openings. This is a large task that can take several days, and traditionally it was undertaken as a particular type of lap labor. Lap labor is a village-based labor system whereby neighbors and relatives take turns helping each other with different domestic and agricultural responsibilities. This reciprocity was important before the cash economy became widespread and is still practiced in many forms of western Sikkim. The center point of the responsibility comes from the relationships between the different residents in a village. Requesting assistance in the form of lap obligates the petitioner to reciprocate and help their neighbor when they have a need. Finding lap laborers has become more complicated since people began finding work outside of the village in the 1980s, a trend abetted by the arrival of tourism in the region and the emphasis on education to attain coveted government jobs. These economic changes have had a significant impact on how people relate to their land and each other, as it is now common for children to go to boarding school and therefore not grow up learning the agricultural cycle and knowledge of the land that comes with it.[8]

BYASU CHADUNG BEYOND COMMODIFICATION

This has impacted the making of different foods, and specifically, snack foods. What happens then when people who are not kin prepare corn, and specifically byasu chadung? In the last decade, this has become increasingly common, and communities have developed creative responses. Since 2018, many members of my family, and others in western Sikkim, have started to order byasu chadung from production teams based in villages around Gyalshing, the district headquarters of the region and the major urban center. The reason for this is time. Increasingly, people feel too busy with professional obligations to take full days to prepare traditional foods. There is often a wait for cartons full of byasu chadung to be delivered, and they are sold for around 2,000 Indian rupees per carton.[9] This is not a small amount of money, and purchasing a carton of commodity snacks, such as Haldirams bhujia mix, Waiwai noodles, or Parle biscuits, is a much cheaper and more convenient option.

However, local community members generally agree that the cultural significance of traditional snacks such as byasu chadung outweighs the cost and convenience factor and therefore, that byasu chadung transcends the status of a commodity. People from different ethnic and religious com-

8. These economic changes are not only taking place in west Sikkim. For broader context in northeast India, see Kikon and Karlsson 2019.

9. This is equivalent to roughly 24 US dollars according to the exchange rate in November 2023.

munities that I talked to about byasu chadung in the summer of 2022 extolled its health benefits, especially for diabetics (diabetes is an increasingly common health issue in western Sikkim); its taste and compatibility with milk tea, the beverage of preference for social engagements in Sikkim; and the distinct aesthetic beauty of the molded, egg-like cups. Mass produced snacks do not taste, look, or smell the same; and as a result, many people told me that these snacks do not facilitate the forging of social relationships in the same way. The continued popularity of byasu chadung, evidenced by the wait for orders in Gyalshing bazaar, demonstrates the continued affection and respect people have for traditional foodways. At the same time, the time-consuming nature of byasu chadung production and specialist knowledge required to make it means its production cannot be usurped by mechanization or mass production. On the one hand, this could make the continued production and consumption of byasu chadung appear tenuous; but, as shown in the last few years in Gyalshing, people are coming up with creative ways to continue to make this food, which means byasu chadung will continue to be enjoyed and will continue to make relations.

PRECIOUS CORN AS FOOD SECURITY AND SOVEREIGNTY

At a time when mass-produced snack foods and agro-industrial corn seeds are easily available, communities in western Sikkim continue to grow crops from heritage seeds and make byasu chadung and other traditional snacks. The time pressures of contemporary life challenge people's ability to do this, but local communities are developing new mechanisms to respond to the continued love for these snacks, including forming production teams that draw on traditional knowledge.

The ubiquitous nature of corn in western Sikkim's agricultural landscape, and its resilience in times of changing weather patterns, has led to the continued use of Kenzong Rinpoche, Precious Corn, as a staple element of Sikkim's food security and sovereignty across different cultural communities. The cultivation and consumption of corn are underpinned by older traditions and systems of knowledge, as are the relations that corn fosters. Corn has long sustained and nourished Sikkim's human communities as well as more-than-human communities in the form of the birds and bears that eat it from the fields and the spirits to whom it is offered in ritual traditions. In Lhopo Buddhist communities, the resilience and versatility of corn is explained by its connection to the position of Sikkim as a Valley of Abundance, filled with positive power affirmed by prophecy. Therefore, even as mass-produced snacks appear on tea trays, byasu chadung remains as an agent and reminder in the making of nourishment across Sikkim's seen and unseen dimensions.

13

A Brief Decolonial History of *Khor* among the Tangkhul Nagas

Taimaya Ragui

EARLY IN THE TWENTIETH CENTURY, Western missionaries, predominantly American Baptist missionaries, prohibited the Tangkhul Nagas[1] from consuming *khor*, their traditional rice beer and primary source of nutrition. This domineering act, I argue, has had long-term consequences for their food system, forcing people to rely on external supplies. As for their social system, the prohibition of *khor*, which was a direct result of the imposition of colonial ideals, caused communal divide during the colonial and postcolonial times. This reality necessitates decolonizing food to reclaim traditional cultures and redeem cultural identity.[2] Decolonization through community action or a community process that would help the Tangkhul Nagas to delink from colonial captivity and reclaim essential cultural values is necessary to address the continuing colonial influence on

1. An Indigenous community that lives in the Indo-Myanmar border districts of Ukhrul and Kamjong, located in the state of Manipur in Northeast India.

2. Dolly Kikon discusses, in a different context, "how fermenting cultures shape citizenship practices and identities" (Kikon 2021, 376).

their contemporary socioreligious realities. This can be achieved by the decolonization of theology, which debunks the imposition of a colonial God, and the decolonization of knowledge to recover forms of knowledge that are relational, experimental, and continuous.

The terms "decolonize" or "decolonization" signify a complex and multifaceted process of transitioning away from colonial power. Over the years, they have broadly been employed as a political and intellectual endeavor. In the former, colonies make an effort to achieve independence from colonial powers and establish self-governance (see Fanon 1966; Hargreaves 1996), whereas the latter seeks to delink or dismantle colonial structures, systems, and ideologies that were enforced by the colonizers (see Smith 1999; Mignolo 2000).[3] In this paper, I use the concept of decolonization to emphasize the necessity to historicize precolonial Tangkhul history and knowledge by using local voices, such as oral tradition (elders) and local writings, rather than exclusively depending on colonial texts (like colonial findings, reports, translation works, and ethnographic works). In addition to referencing written texts, this chapter seeks to capture the voices of mothers and grandmothers who traditionally inherit the skill to brew *khor* and who continue to illicitly brew alcohol today.[4] Occasionally, it will also refer to the voices of fathers and grandfathers to understand the experience and socioreligious reality of *khor* intake.

ARRIVAL AND INFLUENCE OF THE COLONIALS ON *KHOR* CONSUMPTION

In 1890, William Pettigrew came to India, inspired by Adoniram Judson, an early Protestant missionary to Burma. While working for the Arthington Aborigines Mission in Calcutta, he was inspired to relocate to Manipur due to the Anglo-Manipur War of 1891 (Moore et al. 1895, 4–5; see also

---

3. According to David Gardinier, the term "decolonization" initially referred to a political occurrence but subsequently broadened to encompass all aspects of the colonial experience, including those of a political, economic, cultural, and psychological nature (Gardinier 1968, 269).

4. The Manipur cabinet has approved the sale and consumption of liquor in the state (Sept. 2022), although there are objections from women's groups and activists, as well as the church in Christian-dominated areas. Among Indigenous communities, individuals who continue to brew *khor* are frowned upon because the colonists regard it as sinful and immoral.

Stanley 1998, 166–71). Before his arrival, no Western missionaries had been granted access to Manipur, making him the pioneer in spreading the gospel in the region (de St. Dalmas 1894, 3–4). He received permission to enter Manipur with the help of the then-officiating political agent, Alexander Porteous (Singh 1996, 7). However, when the official political agent, Major Patrick Maxwell, returned from furlough, Pettigrew was ordered to cease his ministry in the Manipur valley. Instead, Pettigrew was given the permission to continue his work among the Tangkhul Nagas in the hill areas (Moore et al. 1895, 4–5).

After surveying and recognizing the potential for mission work in Ukhrul, a Tangkhul Naga village, Pettigrew began his work in early 1896 (Pettigrew 1897a, 325; Downs 1971, 79). He came with the notion that his religion and culture were superior, while the local Indigenous ways of life were perceived as inferior. In the words of Walter D. Mignolo's description of colonialism, he arrived with a "coloniality of power," in which colonial ideals are imposed upon Indigenous communities, who are then compelled to adopt them (2000, 17). In fact, in one of Pettigrew's earliest missionary reports, he characterized the Tangkhul Nagas as "uncivilized," "demon worshippers," and "superstitious" (1897, 325). They were also categorized as "animistic in their worship, very superstitious, and addicted to [*khor*] drinking to a great extent" (1899, 50–55). The colonizers made derogatory and condescending remarks about tribal-Indigenous communities, such as the Tangkhul Naga community, in their reports and findings. Tribal-Indigenous communities were portrayed as uncivilized in comparison to European societies, which were used as a standard for measuring the advancement of other ethnic groups (Mandavilli 2019, 26).

This was evident in, among other places, their treatment of alcoholic beverages. For instance, after receiving permission to enter Manipur, Pettigrew fondly recalls his intention to substitute the boxes that previously contained *colonial* alcoholic drinks, "Liqueur Whiskey and Old Silent Malt," with books and clothing (1894, 5).[5] However, he derided the local rice beer, *zu*, which is equivalent to Tangkhul *khor*, in his missionary

5 When asked if they remembered Western missionaries drinking alcohol, some grandmothers could not recall, while others presume that they did.

reports (1899, 50–55). Additionally, according to Arkotong Longkumar, the consumption of or abstinence from rice beer was also used to differentiate genuine converts from nominal ones in Naga contexts (2016, 3). It served as a criterion for determining whether the new converts could adhere to the Christian standard of abstinence.

The civilizing mission (that is, the imposition of Western cultural and religious values) of Tangkhul Nagas began with the imposition of Western education in Ukhrul (Singh 1996, 7–13). This was achieved by establishing a school in 1896 and forcing the Indigenous community to attend (Pettigrew 1897b, 526). After five years of working with them, Pettigrew baptized twelve of his students in 1901 (Shimray n.d., 15). In the following year, a church was built, which is now known as the Phungyo Baptist Church. In the six years that followed, the number of converts reached seventy (Luikham 1948, 22). However, according to T. Luikham, one of the early converts sensed a sense of stagnancy in the practice of the Christian faith, particularly as its numbers grew (23). This stagnation was viewed by Pettigrew as an impasse between those who continue to consume *khor* and those who believe in the truthfulness of the Christian faith. In response, Pettigrew made an attempt in 1907 to reform Tangkhul Christian religious practices by prohibiting *khor* consumption (23). This endeavor to change their culture was met with resistance by the new converts and most of them left the church, with only seven remaining.

This was again followed by a significant church split in March 1908 (Pettigrew 1986, 57). The divide was between those who wanted to be Christians and participate in traditional festivals and those who disassociated their Christian faith from their traditional cultural identity. The conflict stemmed from the participation of new converts in the festival of death known as *thisam phanit*.[6] Pettigrew describes the outcome of this conflict as follows:

> The missionaries fully realising the need of what some will be pleased to call radical measures, called the church together and advised them to settle once for all this question of participation in

6. For detailed discussion of the festival, see Pettigrew 1909, 37–46.

> a feast which included the offering of sacrifice to evil spirits. We fully expected all to lapse back into the heathenism owing to the powerful influence of tribal custom, but seven of thirty-five church members decided to withdraw and form a new church (1986, 57).

Typically, a festival is a gathering of the community with a great deal of *kashak kazā* (food) and *khor*, accompanied by the sacrifice of animals to their Gods and spirits (Horam 1977, 40). Pettigrew, however, saw these Indigenous festivals as "pagan" rituals that offered sacrifices to evil spirits and thus signified an attempt to revert to their traditional-primal religion. Hence, asking them to refrain or, worse, prohibiting an agrarian-communitarian society's participation in festivals would eventually have devastating effects on their food and social systems. This is because the food habits and social life of the Indigenous communities were inextricably linked to their festivities.

Eventually, as colonial ideologies were enforced through the establishment of schools and the planting of churches, participation in cultural festivals associated with traditional religion and the consumption of *khor* became stigmatized, if not criminalized. Furthermore, *khor* consumption or nonconsumption was interpreted as "a way of sifting 'actual' from 'nominal' converts, checking to see if they could meet the new Christian 'standard' of abstinence" (Longkumer 2016, 3). However, throughout the colonial and postcolonial periods, the Tangkhul Nagas had a strong desire to partake in their cultural festivals or events (Horam 1977, 14, 40). The new converts viewed them through the stereotypes of devout believers who forsake traditional festivals and unbelievers who adhere to traditional practices.

This conflict further resulted in a third church-community split in the 1950s, when Roman Catholics arrived in Tangkhul inhabited areas (Jeyaseelan 1996, 69–70). According to Āyi Kong, in addition to receiving food and clothing as gifts, they were given the choice of being permitted to consume *khor* if they decided to join the Roman Catholic Church.[7] When the Indigenous community was given the alternative of being

7. In contemporary Tangkhul, the consumption of any alcoholic beverage is considered immoral, if not a sin. Āyi Kong is eighty-one years old. Āyi Kong, interview, April 2023.

punished for drinking *khor* or joining a new church where they could continue to drink, a considerable number of people chose the latter and left the Baptist church.

THE IMPACT OF *KHOR* PROHIBITION ON THE TANGKHUL FOOD AND SOCIAL SYSTEM

The colonials prohibited new converts from participating in cultural festivals and consuming *khor* for more than one reason. On the surface, it appears that Western missionaries regarded *khor* consumption as an impediment to genuine religious conversion (Longkumer 2016, 8). On a deeper level, however, the prohibition was an expression of the colonial belief of the West's cultural superiority over Indigenous cultures. Just as colonists viewed their religion as superior and believed that it was their mission to save the Indigenous communities from darkness, they also believed that their cuisine was superior and that their whiskey, for instance, was superior to *khor* (Pettigrew 1894, 50–55).

In addition, the Tangkhul Nagas were prohibited from consuming *khor* if they desired to convert to the new faith. Pettigrew used the early converts to enforce this prohibition. Āyi Thing, who is ninety-seven years old and witnessed the work of the first missionaries, vividly recalls the early converts going door-to-door and telling people to stop brewing *khor* and *zam* (rice wine).[8] With this knowledge in mind, this section considers the impact of prohibition of khor consumption on two domains: the food system and the social system.

Food System

The history of the Tangkhul food and economic system can be categorized into three stages: the first reflects the Tangkhul's migratory phase during which they gathered food from the forest; the second reflects their transition from caves to huts and from food gathering to food production; and the third stage is when they began to establish an agrarian community (Shimrei 2016, 14). Western missionaries may have arrived in Ukhrul when the Tangkhuls had reached the third stage of their food system. In

---

8. Āyi Thing is ninety-seven years old. Āyi Thing, interview, May 2023.

those days, while sharing food was a prevalent practice, formal exchange of goods happened through a marketplace barter system called *leingapha* (Vashum 2017, 45–47).

The Tangkhul Nagas are an agricultural community. This means their primary source of food production is agriculture, which is supplemented by hunting, fishing, and herb and fruit gathering (Konghay 2016, 27–28). Their belief in Gods and spirits is inextricably linked to these practices, which involve the natural world. They held a three-tiered understanding of Gods: *Āmeoa* (the Creator), *Zingwungleng* (the God of heavens), and *Kokto* (God/ruler of death). In their agricultural activities, they would pray to *Ā meoa* and *Zingwungleng* for blessings, and they sought to lead a good life in preparation for the next life, which was ruled by *Kokto*. This belief system has profound associations, as their belief in *kameo* (spirit) related to the natural world, such as *shim kameo* (spirit of the house), *kong kameo* (spirit of the river), *lui kameo* (spirit of the field), *ngalung kameo* (spirit of the rock), *kaphung kameo* (spirit of the mountain), and so on (Kharay 2021, 15).

In this faith system, the Tangkhul Naga belief in *Phunghui Philava*, the God/Goddess of wealth, is associated with food production (Thumra 2003, 65). It is believed that the harvest will be abundant if *Phunghui Philava* walks through the paddy field. Thus, Tangkhul Naga people begin the year with a seed-sowing festival known as *Luira Phanit*, in which they pray to *Phunghui Philava* for protection from disaster and a bountiful harvest (Horam 2013, 14). Before colonialism, when they prayed or offered sacrifices to their Gods and deities/spirits, they did so alongside the offering of *khor* and other animal sacrifices.[9] *Khor* was not only a staple food, but also an essential component of their traditional religion. In Christian parlance, khor was used in the worship of Gods. This indicates that Nagas considered it inconceivable to participate in a feast, festival, or celebration without consuming *khor*. In fact, its significance transcends rituals, ceremonies, and social gatherings and extends to their spirituality. According to Āyi Yang, every family used to brew *khor* and were expected to prepare *khor* for special occasions.[10] For example, if there was an upcoming special

9. Āyi Kong interview.

10. Āyi Yang is ninety-three years old. Āyi Yang, interview, May 2023.

family event, the immediate family members and relatives would help prepare *khor* for the occasion. She added that everyone, including men and women, used to drink *khor*. Like the Tangkhul Nagas, other Naga tribes considered rice beer indispensable. Christoph von Furer-Haimendorf, an anthropologist who conducted participant observation research on the Nagas in the 1930s, suggests the following regarding Ao Nagas:

> What wine is to the Italian and whisky to the Scotchman, rice-beer is to the Naga. It refreshes him on hot days, encourages him to carry the heavy harvest-baskets many hundreds of feet up the steep mountains to the village, loosens his tongue, and makes him merry when, on feast days, he sits with his friends round the fire (Furer-Haimendorf 1939, 57).

When the Nagas converted to Christianity and decided to be baptized as a sign of their commitment to Jesus Christ, they were required to give up *khor*, their staple food. In fact, Western missionaries threatened the Ao Nagas with eternal damnation in hell if they did not cease drinking rice beer (57). When *khor* consumption, which consists primarily of rice and was part of their breakfast, lunch, and dinner, was prohibited, there were not many alternatives available.[11] When asked what replaced their staple food, the responses varied. Āyi Kong and Thing think that *khor* was replaced by a nonalcoholic beverage known as *zat thur*[12]; Āyi Shi and Āvā Shim suggest that they drank either plain water or *bikha chā* (black tea).[13] Āva̱ Shon and Āva̱ Shom acknowledge the use of *bikha chā*, but say that *khor/zam* was replaced by *leiyi* (distilled alcohol).[14]

---

11. Indigenous rice beer has a thick texture. Its major ingredients are sticky rice (m nui), water (tara), and thing ngayung (root) or herbs. The sticky rice is pounded, mixed with water, and seasonings are added to create a thick texture with a fermented flavor. A study on the nutritional content of rice beer showed it is nutritionally rich and has medicinal value (Bhuyan et al. 2014, 142–48).

12. Āyi Kong interview; Āyi Thing interview.

13. Āyi Shi is ninety-six, while Āvā Shim is seventy-four years old. Āyi Shi, interview, May 2023; Āvā Shim, interview, May 2023.

14. Āva̱ Shon, interview, May 2023; Āva̱ Shom, interview, May 2023.

Zat thur had a place in Christian households, but its similarity to *khor* and lack of alcoholic content prevented it from gaining popularity. Although it is still prepared in some households, it is no longer considered a staple food. The successful replacement of *khor* with *bikha chā* came at a cost. Tuisem Ngakang argues that the Western missionaries' substitution of *khor* with *bikha chā* represented their greatest act of cultural imperialism (Ngakang 2022, 306). The nutritional value of *bikha chā* is inferior to that of *khor*, and the ingredients for *bikha chā* (i.e., tea leaf and sugar) must be purchased with money (Ngakang 2022, 306; Furer-Haimendorf 1939, 57). I would add that this shift implicitly sowed the seeds of capitalism. Except for salt, the Tangkhuls had a self-sufficient food system. Although they could harvest salt in some Tangkhul villages, they previously imported salt from Myanmar's Indigenous tribal communities (Lungleng 2011, 20). However, they then had to begin importing sugar and tea from other parts of the country. Consequently, colonizers instilled the necessity of relying on others for economic needs, thereby affecting the Indigenous food system.

In addition to affecting the food system, the displacement of *khor* with *leiyi* impacted the health of Tangkhuls. *Khor* consumption is associated with longevity and good health, whereas drinking *leiyi* is associated with serious health hazards. The prohibition of brewing *khor* and the Manipur state's eventual decision to remain a dry state led to illicit selling of *leiyi*, as well as health hazards, such as liver and kidney diseases.[15] For example, there have been instances of people being harmed after consuming unregulated *leiyi* or other locally produced distilled alcohol.[16]

Social System

In the context of the Tangkhul Nagas, a person's identity was traditionally linked to his or her family, clans, or village, and their shared cultural activities.

15. Ninglun Hanghal, "Storm in A Bottle: The Story of Prohibition in Manipur," *Tatsat Chronicles*, November 18, 2022.

16. This argument is used to repeal alcohol prohibition. Rokibuz Zaman, "High and Dry: Why the Dilution of Manipur's Widely Flouted Liquor Ban Has Sparked Protests," *Scroll*, October 21, 2022; (see also Chonchuirinmayo Luithui, "Who Killed the Rice Beer?" *Kangla Online*, August 29, 2014).

Prior to colonization, their religious and cultural practices were interconnected (Vashum 2003, 68). There was no distinct religious identity in the sense that we understand it today. The introduction of Christianity by Western missionaries was accompanied by the propagation of a dualistic style of thinking. It begins with referring to those who have not yet heard the Christian gospel as "unreached."[17] This dualistic worldview is manifested in further binaries: White and others, civilized and uncivilized, believers and nonbelievers, etc. In the Tangkhul Naga context, after the dissemination of the gospel by Western missionaries, the larger community was divided into those who had been baptized and those who had not, those who had relocated to the new village and those who remained in the old village, Baptists and Roman Catholics, etc. These classifications were also centered on the distinction between *khor* drinkers and non-*khor* drinkers.

When some Tangkhul Nagas adopted the new faith, they experienced pushback from family members, relatives, and villagers. In some cases, they were compelled to leave their homes; there were also cases where adherents of the traditional religion threatened or persecuted the new converts (Luikham 1948, 34). This was one of the community's earliest instances of socioreligious conflict. Moreover, as noted above, they were forced to embrace colonial values. In the long run, this had a ripple effect in terms of denomination-based community division. The division of the Tangkhul Naga community along denominational lines would breed deep mistrust within the community, particularly among Tangkhul Baptists and Catholics. For example, as Roman Catholics emerged among the Tangkhul Nagas as a result of their separation from Baptists, and as they continued to permit alcohol consumption, Baptist Tangkhuls looked down on their professed spirituality as Christians. In addition to creating distrust within the Tangkhul community, the prohibition of *khor* resulted in the loss of a social skill (namely, brewing *khor*) and the demise of cultural events associated with *khor* (such as *Thisam Phanit*).

The colonial legacy of *khor* prohibition continues to reverberate in the present. I conducted interviews with multiple Tangkhul Naga *āva̱ngarā*

17. This category was used to strategize Pettigrew's mission approach (Dena, n.d.:1).

(mothers) and *āyingarā* (grandmothers) to ask them about the state of *khor* consumption and production today. When *āvangarā* and *āyingarā* who illicitly brew *leiyi* (distilled alcohol) are asked about these concerns, they are confident that they will be able to brew *khor* again, especially if they have the traditional pot for brewing it. However, they are concerned that the younger generation will lack traditional skills and have neglected several cultures.[18] They are concerned because brewing *khor* was a social and life skill learned from their *āvangarā* and *āyangarā*.

In addition, my conversations with mothers and grandmothers showed that those who illicitly brew *zam* or *leiyi* are stigmatized and regarded as social outcasts. In today's Tangkhul context, a handful of people still brew *khor* and *zam* for personal consumption, while *leiyi* is made for commercial use. Those who do so are stigmatized or placed on the margins of society. Āva̱ Ngam, a fifty-six-year-old mother who makes a living by producing *leiyi*, believes they are mistreated by society.[19] Due to an ill-conceived understanding of *khor* or *leiyi* consumption, she feels obligated to make restitution to the society. She adds that whenever she attends a church service, she feels as if the sermon is specifically targeted at her because preachers condemn alcohol consumption and production. While Āva̱ Won is uncertain about how others perceive her or her family, when she is out and about in society, she feels "ashamed of herself."[20] Even though people do not directly confront her, she and her family are treated poorly in society, particularly at church gatherings. Āyi Pung, a former brewer of *khor* and *zam*, does not wish to attend social gatherings or church services due to the unfair treatment she receives.[21] The prohibition of local liquors during the colonial period thus continues to influence how people view those who consume or produce liquor: they are stigmatized and regarded as the worst sinners.

18. Āyi Chung is ninety, while Āyi Pung is eighty-plus years old (unsure of her age). Āyi Chung, interview, May 2023; Āyi Pung, interview, May 2023.

19. Āva Ngam, interview, May 2023.

20. Āva̱ Won, interview, May 2023.

21. Ayi Pung interview.

DECOLONIZING FOOD

The brief history of *khor* and its prohibition presented here underscores the deep connection between (colonial) theology and the consumption and colonial prohibition of Indigenous foodways. I thus think that decolonizing food among the Tangkhul Nagas necessitates decolonizing theology and knowledge. Decolonizing theology means debunking the imposition of a colonial God and its juxtaposition to a traditional God, while decolonizing knowledge means recovering a form of knowledge that is relational, experimental, and continual. Decolonizing theology, I propose, should take the form of analyzing how colonizers brought their God view, how they perceived the Indigenous God, and then how they began reconstructing tribal-Indigenous understandings of God, who have now mostly converted to Christianity. The colonizers brought a dualistic understanding of God and the God world, separating the sacred from the secular. Thus, they believed that Indigenous people had a two-tiered conception of God (Eaton 1984, 52, 54). In this narrow view of the tribal-Indigenous God, the Supreme Being or Creator is distant from humanity and the natural world. The colonists thought that tribal-Indigenous communities only interacted with *kameo* or spirits through sacrifices or offerings. Consequently, when tribal-Indigenous communities participated in festivals and offered meat and *khor*, it was perceived as meat and *khor* being offered to *kameo*; they were also labeled as animistic since their practices were perceived as uncivilized, heathen, superstitious, demon worship, and the like (Thomas 2016, 54). However, a closer examination of their traditional religion reveals that they held a three-tiered view of God the Creator (*Āmeoa*), the God of the heavens (*Zingwungleng*), and the God/ruler of death (*Kokto*) (Khongreiwo 2011, 43–67; Kharay 2021, 1–21). This is meant to imply that Tangkhuls had a high view of God and the God world that could guide their decisions, as well as the larger Christian community's discussion of God talk. Because the prohibition of *khor* consumption emerged out of a narrow, colonialist view of God, this task of decolonizing theology would help in debunking colonial misconceptions, help in reconsidering their narrative about God and God talk. In doing so, it would help the tribal-Indigenous community in beginning to engage in the task of decolonial theology, that is, reconstructing their view of God.

In turn, the decolonization of theology might help lift the stigma around *khor* consumption and production and reopen access to the Indigenous foodways of the Tangkhul Naga people.

To advance the decolonial tasks, I would further suggest the need to understand knowledge sharing among Tangkhul Nagas (Ragui, 2023). Knowledge was what the community knew, believed, and practiced within different subsections of society. For example, knowledge is knowing that their livelihood is dependent on the soil/land and believing that their Gods and spirits watch over them; therefore, food items, such as *khor* and meat, are offered to please their Gods/spirits and to bestow abundant blessings upon them (Horam 1977, 39). Informally, they learn life skills by observing their parents and relatives; formally, they learn social and life skills through their traditional education system, known as *longshim*. The knowledge that they acquire in longshim prepares them for life in the community, village, and beyond. However, because Western missionaries associated *longshim* and the consumption of *khor* during feasts with heathenism, Tangkhul people were also forced to abandon these practices (Furer-Haimendorf 1939, 56). Knowledge is passed on to the next generation through the platforms of school and church, but it is devoid of Indigenous people's traditional knowledge. The perception of "knowledge" is now cognitive or text-based, and it is predominantly indicated by English literacy. Oral tradition has been supplanted by the written education system and print culture (Kharingpam 2020, 1). In contrast, Indigenous conceptions of knowledge are: relational, as young people learn from elders, including parents, grandparents, relatives, and village elders; experimental, as they experiment and acquire various life skills at *longshim*, until they decide to marry; and continuous, as what they learn in *longshim* will be applied in their everyday, community, and village life. Furthermore, rather than being limited to restricted curriculum-based lessons, their education was vibrant and entrenched in their community and village life.

CONCLUSION

This chapter aimed to decolonize food, particularly *khor*, by examining how colonials imposed their ideologies and diminished the Tangkhul Nagas' traditional cultures. As a result of prohibiting the consumption of *khor* without understanding its significance, colonists exerted a deep, negative impact on the Tangkhul food system and social system. Prior to the arrival of Western missionaries, *khor* was used to offer sacrifices to Gods and spirits; after their arrival, *khor* consumption became synonymous with immorality. To delink the Tangkhul Nagas from colonial captivity, theology and knowledge must be decolonized. This is said in the expectation that such decolonization work will enable the Tangkhul Nagas to engage in community action, both to debunk colonial ideologies and to reclaim and redeem their traditional cultures and identities.

SECTION V

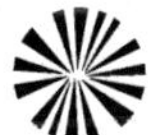

SOUTHEAST ASIA

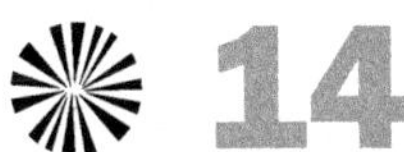

The *Thingification* of Palm Oil
The Machine, Its Masters, and Its Menace

Lynnette Xiangling Li

When I grew up in Singapore, the monsoon winds brought the smell of smoke from the distant burning forests of Kalimantan and Sumatra in Indonesia. During the time of writing this chapter, the air quality in Singapore has fallen to unhealthy levels.[1] This perennial problem is brought about by smoke from fires in Indonesia caused by slash-and-burn tactics to clear land to make way for monocrop cultivation—in particular, palm trees to produce palm oil. While the burning of forests to expand palm plantations may seem like a distant and isolated matter, its impact was omnipresent with each inhalation of air that smelled like burnt wood. In addition to the worsening air quality, the smoke-induced haze blocked out the sunshine, creating a dark, ominous feeling compounded by the advice that people remain indoors.

1. Chen Lin, "Haze Hits Singapore as Hot Spots in Indonesia's Sumatra Increase," *Reuters*, October 7, 2023.

In hazy conditions, Singaporeans have the option to close their windows and rely on their air-conditioning units to give them respite from the smell of distant burning embers. Indeed, Cherian George, a political commentator, has referred to Singapore as an "air-conditioned city," critiquing it as a "society with a unique blend of comfort and central control, where people have mastered their environment, but at the cost of individual autonomy, and at the risk of unsustainability" (George 2020, 19). The privilege of living in air-conditioned silos while the air outside is unhealthy has a connection to dignity, as sociologist Teo You Yenn reminds us that "dignity is like clean air" in that "you do not notice its absence unless it is in short supply" (Teo 2019, 202). The dignity of clear air is something Indonesians living within the vicinity of burning forests are denied, and many do not have the privilege of running air-conditioning units to take sanctuary from the thick haze of smoke.

The slash-and-burn methods of clearing land to expand palm plantations begins the process of palm oil production in Indonesia and in some cases in Malaysia. The palm oil production process finds its way back to Singapore, where the world's largest palm oil refinery is located. The interconnectedness of the production of palm oil reflects the different parts of the machinery of domination, submission, control, and manipulation of resources—land, water, and people. The machinery, masters, and menace of palm oil have been weaponized to the detriment of the quality of life for many in southeast Asia.

This chapter draws upon Aimé Césaire's concept of *thingification* in his influential work *Discourse on Colonialism*. The process of *thingification* is about the domination and submission of those who are colonized. This includes the resources of land, water, and labor. At the heart of colonization is what Césaire calls *thingification*, a process whereby those who are colonized are turned into "instruments of production" (and, one might add, instruments *for* production). He defines the concept:

> Between colonizer and colonized there is room only for forced labor, intimidation, pressure, the police, taxation, theft, rape, compulsory crops, mistrust, arrogance, self-complacency, swinishness,

> brainless elites, degraded masses. No human contact, but relations of domination and submission which turn the colonizing man into a classroom monitor, an army sergeant, a prison guard, a slave driver, and the indigenous man into an instrument of production. My turn to state an equation: colonization = "thingification" (2000, 42).

Thingification is enmeshed with colonization, and Césaire reminds us that "no one colonizes innocently" (36). This is exactly why, for Césaire, the process of colonization makes objects out of people, natural resources, and systems. Instead of being treated with intrinsic dignity as the *beings* that they are, their value to the colonial project is their utility, monetary profitability, and control over socio-economic networks. The colonization process manufactures docility amongst its subjects into subordination to its powers of organization. They are things subjected to being owned, manipulated, extracted, and made inanimate. They are *thingified*.

Monocrop plantations are often justified through the rhetoric of progress through development. However, this rhetoric ultimately serves to divert power towards those invested in the colonial project. In this case, it is that of the palm plantations. The rhetoric of progress shapes the attitudes and ethos around social and economic development. It alters the social consciousness and structural positioning of those whose lives, cultures, traditions, and lands are consumed into the project of palm oil plantations. Leonardo and Clodovis Boff question the efficacy of such "developments" and who stands to benefit from them. They remind us that such "development" positioned as progress functions to "benefit only some strata of the population, marginalizing broader sectors" (1988, 6). Environmental philosopher Seyyed Hossein Nasr cautions that when nature becomes a "thing," it is "devoid of meaning, and at the same time the void created by the disappearance of this vital aspect of human existence continues to live within the souls of men and to manifest itself in many ways, sometimes violently and desperately" (1997, 17). Hence, this chapter analyzes the intersectional ways in which the production of palm oil has been *thingified* to look at the power dynamics behind its machine, masters, and contribution as menace.

THE USES OF PALM OIL IN FOOD PRODUCTION

Palm oil is cheap, shelf-stable, and readily available and has multiple uses in food production. These qualities have led to not only the rising dependency on palm oil, but also an exorbitant rise for its demand. The use of palm oil in the manufacturing of food often goes unnoticed. Yet, at the same time, the use of palm oil for food manufacturing is virtually impossible to avoid. On the one hand, palm oil is inconspicuous to the average consumer. On the other, palm oil's use is unavoidable. In 2016, roughly 70 percent of palm oil in the United States was used in food production or sold as cooking oil.[2] The production and demand for palm oil is on the rise globally. In 2022–2023, 78 million metric tons were produced, marking a substantial increase from the 58.9 million metric tons produced in the 2015–2016 crop year.[3] Additionally, the demand in palm oil production has been exacerbated due to the invasion of Ukraine, which is a primary producer of a common vegetable oil, namely sunflower oil.[4] This adversely affects ecology, economy, and social equity in detrimental ways. In the past decade, corporations that monopolize the palm oil industry have touted palm oil as the greener vegetable oil substitute. This narrative is heavily contested. At best, it is a form of greenwashing. We must unmask and uncover the realities of the *thingification* of palm oil production because the process of producing palm oil is intrinsically colonial.

THE MACHINERY: CORPORATE OCCUPATION

Plantations were the bedrock of European colonial expansion in Asia and Africa (Murray-Li and Semedi 2021, 1). Profits extracted from plantations in colonies contributed to significant economic gains for colonial empires. In a similar fashion, the coloniality of palm oil plantations is manifested

---

2. "Estimated market share of palm oil in the United States in 2016 and 2022, by application," Statista, https://www.statista.com/statistics/883763/us-palm-oil-market-share-by-type/.

3. "Production volume of palm oil worldwide from 2012/13 to 2023/24," Statista, https://www.statista.com/statistics/613471/palm-oil-production-volume-worldwide/.

4. "The War in Ukraine Is Rocking the Market for Edible Oils: Consumer-Goods Giants Risk Going Hungry," *The Economist*, May 7, 2022.

in their control by corporations.[5] These corporations take on colonial and imperialistic ideology of dominance for political economy in the guise of job creation, climate mitigation, and sustainable development (Murray-Li and Semedi, 7, 9, 57–61). Corporations controlling palm oil plantations are an occupying force in their strategies and usurping tactics to dominate and domesticate land towards the cultivation and extraction of palm oil through monoculture agriculture. This exploitation is corporate occupation at work. This is the machinery of dominance.

The establishment of palm oil plantations, mills to extract palm oil, and ways to sell, market, and transport palm oil did not happen overnight. Instead, it was done little by little, taking away of land from its original inhabitants, luring migrants from other Indonesian regions, and training workers that contribute to an intersecting machinery of plantocracy. Palm oil as a cash crop is dependent on the *thingification* of people, land, and water. They become objects of a process that contributes toward goals of profitability. This creeping process of *thingification* is done little by little, inching away at every opportunity it gets. As this form of occupation is gradual, the messaging of progress and development through palm plantations is etched in the hearts of the people to get them on board with a hopeful vision of a more prosperous and progressive society. For countries such as Malaysia and Indonesia, palm oil plantations are pimped as icons of modernity, progress, and national prosperity. These plantations are touted as solutions for job creation and "wasted" land by developing it into a productive, efficient contributor to local economies. At the same time, this development program repeats colonial tropes that consider natives and locals of the land to be poor landowners who fail to fully maximize the utility of their land.

In Tania Murry-Li and Pujo Semedi's ethnographic work, *Plantation Life in Indonesia's Oil Palm Zone*, this pervasive attitude regarding the lazy native is seen in how Sumatran plantation managers would treat workers as if they were "unruly children in need of firm guidance" (2021, 85). This was the colonial legacy of plantation life in Sumatra that Ann Stoler

5. Jonathan Robins, "Shallow Roots: The Early Oil Palm Industry in Southeast Asia, 1848–1940," Journal of Southeast Asian Studies 51, no. 4 (December 2020): 539.

highlights in her article "Perceptions of Protest": plantation managers would typecast their workers as "child-like, vulnerable, and all the more 'dangerous' because of their political susceptibility" (1985, 653). The need to treat workers in a paternalistic fashion, according to Stoler, was to protect them from being easily "conned" (653). The colonial caricature of plantation workers or laborers as ill-disciplined, unthinking, and lazy functions to infantilize them. This perpetuates what Syed Hussein Alatas writes about in his seminal book *The Myth of the Lazy Native*, which highlights how ruling powers of colonial capitalism accentuate how "the degradation of the native population could be considered as a historical necessity" for them to later "accept a subordinate place in the scheme of things" (1977, 24), thereby creating a power hierarchy differentiating the owners, managers, and workers. The infantilization of workers implies that workers lacked the intellectual and emotional maturity, as well as agency. Hence the need to be treated in paternalistic ways. This is part of the *thingification* process. It "thingifies" people into mere laborers devoid of agency and intellect.

Such justifications are prevalent, accepted, and normalized to praise palm oil plantations as a salvific means for local populations to escape poverty and underdeveloped infrastructure. As social ethicist Miguel De La Torre puts it, the "occupation of our minds is more insidious than the occupation of our lands, for if it is our minds (that) are occupied, then the very physical and metaphysical essence of our being becomes subjugated to domination" (2022, 7). Under this machinery of corporate-colonial occupation, local residents are conscripted into modernizing and have to give up their land, livelihoods, and culture for the occupation of palm oil corporations on the promise of trickle-down economic prosperity and progress.

ITS MASTERS: OWNERS FROM BEYOND AND WITHIN

When it comes to the ownership of palm oil plantations, there are owners who are seen and unseen as the power of ownership of capital, land, and the control of labor is distributed very differently. The major stakeholders and ownership of the corporations that own palm plantations and its manufacturing industry are linked to the wealthy merchant class of Malaysia, Indonesia, and Singapore, whose fortunes benefited from colonial era wealth.[6] Companies such as the Sime Darby Berhad can trace their roots to the colonial era. Kumpulan Guthrie Berhad's history goes back to 1821, "as a trading company and as agents for twelve British companies with plantations in what was then Malaya" (Teoh 2012, 22).

Although Singapore, my country of birth, does not have any palm oil plantations within its geographical boundaries, it plays a pivotal role in raising capital through initial public offerings (IPOs) and listings on the Singapore (Stock) Exchange. It has done so since the late 1990s for several plantation-based companies. Singapore and various international banks such as Rabobank provide secure funding for the expansion of palm oil industry in Indonesia (Teoh 2012, 33). Apart from the capital raising towards palm oil plantation expansion, Singapore is where one of the world's largest oil plantation owners, Wilmar International, is based. As of December 2022, Wilmar International owns more than 231,697 hectares of planted area, of which 65 percenet are in Indonesia and 26 percent in east Malaysia.[7] Wilmar International is the world's leading palm oil production company. In 2022, their palm oil market capitalization amounted to 2.02 billion US dollars.[8] Another major stakeholder controlling 1 percent of the global refined and processed palm oil market is Musim Mas. They own more than 130,000 hectares of plantation land in Indonesia.[9] Musim Mas is also headquartered in Singapore.

---

6. Rahmawati Retno Winarni and Jan Willem Van Gelder, "'Tycoon-Controlled Oil Palm Groups in Indonesia'—Executive Summary" (TUK Indonesia and Profundo, 2015), 2–4, https://www.tuk.or.id/wp-content/uploads/2015/02/Tycoons-in-the-Indonesian-palm-oil-sector-140828-Tuk-Summary.pdf.

7. Wilmar International, "Plantation: Oil Palm Plantation and Milling" (Singapore, n.d.), https://www.wilmar-international.com/our-businesses/plantation/oil-palm-plantation-milling#.~:text=Wilmar%20is%20one%20of%20the,Malaysia%20and%209%25%20in%20Africa.

8. "Leading palm oil companies worldwide in 2022, based on market capitalization," https://www.statista.com/statistics/477252/leading-global-plam-oil-companies-based-on-market-capitalization/

9. Nana Shibata, "Singapore-Based Indonesia Palm Oil Exporter Grapples with EU Law," *Asia Nikkei*, October 18, 2023.

Public perception of plantation owners is mixed. On the one hand, plantation owners are seen as usurpers of land by using their political influence to displace villages to acquire more land to expand their plantations through privatization.[10] They would politically organize, rapidly industrialize, and strategically monopolize the palm oil market to dictate its demand, supply, and production (Murray-Li and Semedi, 123–25). Their sole intent is geared toward expansion and profit-making. On the other hand, plantation owners are also seen by the locals as benevolent occupiers who promise urbanization, development, and economic progress for the rural population (9). Plantation corporations contribute to building local infrastructure, roads, and schools. This helps to bolster their image from that of an occupying power to that of a charitable and benevolent force that contributes to elevating the standard of living in rural and indigenous communities (167–68). Plantation corporation owners are praised for being the harbinger of social and economic progress by introducing new ways of living through technology, employment, and even education.

Then there are those bureaucrats within the plantations who are known as the "*orang perusahaan*," which means "company men." These are the masters from within who were recruited through nepotism—often village leaders employed to be "instruments of (plantation) occupation" (Murray-Li and Semedi 2021, 44). They are the plantation managers who are tasked with the daily management of the plantations. They were tasked to create subjects out of workers—disciplined, obedient, submissive, and productive. They face constant pressure to assemble a disciplined labor force as cheap, efficient, and productive. Their justification for their complicity is their ability to enrich themselves and afford motorbikes and satellite televisions. At the same time, these company men end up being ostracized by their neighbors and face fractured or damaged social relationships.

Within Indonesia, the oversupply of labor due to transmigrant workers moving to palm plantations as transient workers allowed plantation

---

10. Jonathan E. Robins, *Oil Palm: A Global History* (Chapel Hill: University of North Carolina Press, 2021), 144.

managers to view labor as disposable. The oversupply of labor also meant workers were eager to please plantation managers and tolerate harsh work conditions to secure their livelihood. Without trade unions for plantation workers, exploitation and abuse of workers remain unchallenged and are enabled. There is exploitation at all levels. This machinery and its insatiable greed have to be appeased and fed. Little by little, the dependency on the interconnecting systems of plantation increases because *all* is centered on the production and profitability of palm oil. And the monoculture agricultural growing of palm oil has its risks, not just financial ones, but social and environmental risks as well.

ITS MENACE: SOCIAL AND ENVIRONMENTAL IMPACTS

Palm oil cultivation and production contribute to the degradation of the environment, natural habitat, and inhabitants. The rising demand for palm oil has increased the rate of deforestation. It has caused an increased demand for plantation expansion, leading to thousands of hectares of land being cleared through mostly the slash and burn method in Central, West, and Southern Kalimantan and Sumatra. The smoke from the forest fires causes haze, which significantly deteriorates air quality, affecting neighboring countries like Malaysia, Singapore, the south of Thailand and at its worse reaching even the Philippines.[11] As a result, biodiversity and animal habitats become casualties of palm oil's insatiable need to expand. The cultivation and production of palm oil severely strain and pollute local water resources as chemical pesticides and fertilizers are used to ensure high crop yield. Plantation workers are consistently exposed to these chemicals. Even with recommendations to provide masks and gloves to reduce harm to workers, the exposure to toxic chemicals is so prevalent in their environment that the efficacy of masks and gloves is questioned. The quality of life for plantation workers, and the viable habitats for displaced animals, is concerning. Noting the harms is one thing. Challenging the systemic oppression or thingification of palm oil plantations is another.

---

11. "Indonesia Haze: Why Do Forests Keep Burning?" *BBC*, September 16, 2019.

CONCLUDING THOUGHTS—SEDIKIT SEDIKIT, LAMA LAMA, JADI BUKIT

Sedikit sedikit, lama lama, jadi bukit is a Malay proverb that my mother would say to me to encourage me to stay the course during tough times. It is often used to remind the listener not to despise the littlest of things. For it is through the process of little by little, "sedikit, sedikit," where one accumulates something that would eventually amount to something great like a mountain, "*lama lama jadi bukit.*" This proverb is an attempt to offer hope—perhaps false hope—reminding one to persevere and stay the course. It functions as a reminder that somehow, the little things matter. Perhaps it is the little things of coins saved, which accumulate into dollars and those in turn slowly accumulate towards a mountain of wealth. It is also a way to maintain tenacity and drive to be patient, keep hustling, and to bear with hardship—which is normalized as necessary. For ultimately, bit by bit, little by little, the sacrifice and perseverance will eventually pay off.

I was taught that "*sedikit sedikit, lama lama, jadi bukit*" was how to work towards accomplishing that which seems impossible. This, however, assumes that there is equal opportunity and meritocracy. This is only a reality for those who benefit from these systems. The myth of meritocracy and progress hinges on these sentiments that if you work hard and apply yourself, you can get ahead. Anyone can get ahead. Anyone can overcome poverty. It is false hope that the systems are not rigged or that there is no preferential treatment towards the powerful, elite, politically connected, and wealthy. It also implies that a person who is in predicament of poverty is poor because of the lack of determination, agency, and resolve. This blames the poor for being poor without taking to consideration of the predatory systems that create the conditions which they are wrestling to survive. This rhetoric resonates with the colonial consciousness that places demand for all that have been *thingified* to have faith in the progress and development that plantations will ultimately bring.

Yet when it comes to the promise of development and progress, the sentiments of "*sedikit sedikit, lama lama, jadi bukit*" resonate from a distance. It is the promise by corporations of palm oil plantations in Malaysia and Indonesia to locals, to those who had depended on the land for generations upon generations. And again, I reiterate that plantations are intrinsically colonial. Palm oil plantations are no different. The establishment of palm plantations, mills to extract palm oil, and ways to sell, market, and transport palm oil did not happen overnight. It is this little by little taking away of land from its original inhabitants, luring of migrants from other Indonesian regions, and training of workers that contribute to an intersecting machinery of plantocracy. Palm oil as a cash crop is dependent on the *thingification* of people, land, and water resources. Aimé Césaire's framing of colonization as thingification allows for us to interrogate ways palm oil plantations establish, build, and maintain oppressive geopolitical and socio-economic structures. The *thingification* of palm oil is a civilizing and domesticizing project that promises progress, development, and prosperity for all. In reality, some have benefitted much more than others.

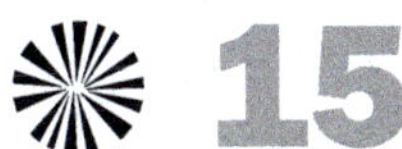 15

Food Colonization, Migration, and Capitalism
A Call to the Batak's Practice of *Marsiadapari*

Hesron H. Sihombing

For many Indigenous communities, food signifies extensive meanings beyond human consumption and survival. It often marks their cultural and communal identity, as what they eat "informs 'who and what they are, to themselves and to others'" (Colás et al. 2022, 5). When European colonizers came and occupied Indigenous lands, they created systems of oppression that included the systematic management of food's production, distribution, and consumption to support colonial structures and protect their interests. In this way, colonization of people and land is inherently connected to what may be called "food colonialism."

I define food colonialism as the structural control, management, appropriation, and distribution of food resources by colonial power for the sake of exerting and expanding colonial dominance upon the colonized people and nature. While the production and management of food resources are important supporting features of the colonial power, food colonialism is not just a means to provide sustenance for the colonizers or generate profit or economic surplus vital to fund the colonial systems or states. Food colonialism also materializes as an inherent tool in the process of colonization itself that is used to exert control, allocate resources for more expansive domination, and subjugate Indigenous communities and their social, cultural, economic, and political subjectivity. Food is weaponized in ways that enable colonization to pierce through the deep tissues of Indigenous culture, worldview, economy, and space/land.

Before the arrival of Dutch colonizers, rice held significance for the Toba Batak people as a "spirit amplifier" that brought forth the sense of community in its production. The Toba Batak people centered rice production around communal planting and harvesting practices called *marsiadapari*. The implementation of the colonial regime of taxation, plantation-style agriculture, and massive migration destroyed this culture by transforming rice into a commodity to be sold on the market. This practice undermines the foundations of the communal practice of *marsiadapari* and thus subjugates the Indigenous subjectivity and worldview of the Toba Batak people.

THE COLONIZATION OF THE BATAK PEOPLE, FOOD COLONIALISM, AND MIGRATION

This chapter addresses food colonialism in the Batak community of Sumatra Island in western Indonesia. The Batak community has six ethnic subgroups: the Toba Batak, Simalungun, Karo, Pakpak, Mandailing, and Angkola. This chapter focuses on the Toba Batak ethnic group, to which I belong. Toba Batak people are the largest group among these six groups; they are predominantly Christians by religion and Lutherans by denomination.

Before the Dutch colonized the Batak land in the mid-nineteenth century, the Batak people had a subsistence and community-based economy. Mainly consisting of mountainous areas and some plateau regions with alluvial land, the Batakland's most fertile sites were on the shores of Lake Toba, Samosir Island, the southern coasts around Balige, and the high valleys of Silindung, which had a large sawah (wet paddy-field) area. Other areas were covered by primeval forests and human settlements (villages) with ladang (dry rice fields) in their surroundings (Kozok 1991, 31–32). The Batak people eat rice as their staple food, alongside maize and tuber cassava. They mastered traditional irrigation systems using wooden pipes in cooperation with neighboring villages. Harvesting took place once a year. The amount of harvest would depend on the quality of irrigation and land conditions.

Fertilization was done with cattle dung and earth from local livestock of pigs, dogs, or chickens (32). The Batak villages had an independent and sustainable economy and provided enough food for everyone. Other needs could be bought in open-air markets held regularly throughout the month.

Christian missionaries from the Rhenish Missionary Society (*Rheinische Missionsgesellschaft, RMG*) came to the Toba Batak land earlier than the Dutch colonizers. The arrival of Ingwer Ludwig Nommensen in Sumatra in 1862 marked the massive conversion of the Toba Batak people to Christianity. Nommensen settled in Silindung Valley of the southern Batak area and began his Batak mission work there. Although he initially faced many difficulties, he finally converted the Toba Batak to Christianity by approaching the local chiefs. Their conversion led their followers and clans to embrace the Christian faith. Mission work continued to expand to other Toba Batak regions, leading to most Toba Batak people becoming Christians. During this regional expansion, the colonial influence initiated and became expedient and paramount to the mission's success.

The overall purpose of Dutch colonialism in the East Indies was not to create new European settlements but to extract resources for surplus through an agricultural system called the "Dutch Cultivation System" (*Cultuurstelsel*), which was implemented from 1830 to 1870. The system required the local people to provide a portion of agricultural products in replacement of and whose amount was equal to the land taxes. The types of agricultural products were usually designated by the colonial government to be profitable for the export market. The amount to surrender to the government was two-fifths of the harvest or in exchange one-fifth of the local's annual work time.[1] This system in Java Island alone generated over one-third of the Dutch government's revenue at its peak and contributed prominently to the Dutch economic growth in the first half of the nineteenth century.[2] Concerning the taxes, about 90 percent of its

1. Sartono Kartidirdjo, *Pengantar Sejarah Baru Indonesia: Sejarah Pergerakan Nasional, Dari Kolonialisme sampai Nasionalisme Jilid* 2 (Jakarta: Gramedia Pustaka Utama, 2014), 15.

2. Melissa Dell and Benjamin A. Olken, "The Development Effects of the Extractive Colonial Economy" in *The Review of Economic Studies*, January 2020, 87, no. 1 (312) (January 2020), 165.

export taxes in the whole East Indies relied on Indigenous agriculture. Therefore, colonial Indonesia's export economy was instrumental to the overall economy of the Dutch (Manse 2022, 414).

However, Uli Kozok, a scholar of Batak history and language, notes that the initial purpose of the colonial annexation of Batakland was not primarily economic, but political. The land was unsuitable for mass production, unlike in the Simalungun and Karo areas, where the plantation economy proliferated (Kozok 1991, 35). Upon the request of RMG missionaries made before Christmas in 1868, the Dutch agreed to colonize the Batakland (Kozok 2010, 22). The colonizers had already occupied the southern borders of the Toba Batak land as early as 1838 (Pelzer 1978, 8), yet they had not formally entered and colonized the Toba Batak land. The main reason for the occupation of the Batakland was to protect it from the military and religious expansion of the Padri Moslem group. This group came from south of the Batak land and had initially converted most of the Mandailing and Angkola Batak people to Islam. The colonial annexation of the land marked the beginning of structural and cultural changes in Batak society.

In non–Toba Batak areas, the Dutch colonizers started to sell the lands through concessions to European planters, including fallow forest land, primeval forest land, and grassland. Karl Pelzer describes the beginning of the plantation process as follows, "The trees were cut; usable timber was saved; everything else was burned" (1978, 46). The colonial administration allotted seventy-five-year land concessions to companies from Europe and the United States. The concessions were regulated based on Western property law. The law ordered sanctions against entities that illegally added more lands beyond what the concessions regulated (Cunningham 1958, 87). By 1890, the planters had complete control of the land except for the land located within the local villages. The local people had no control over the forest land and its conversion to tobacco farms and were not allowed to plant wet rice (Pelzer 2010, 49–50). A Batak village (*huta*) had formerly consisted of the village, rice fields, and the open untouched forest space. The Batak people would leave some forest areas untouched for preservation. They could be used for limited purposes, but only after a community meeting had agreed upon it (Sihombing 2023, 49).

A village functions at once as a religious, political, economic, ecological, and cultural space. A village brings together the interrelationships of humans, God, and nature (Sihombing 2023, 48). Still, when the Dutch colonizers and European planters came, they demarcated the villages to exclude the forest and some rice fields before they were used for their extractive plantations. The colonizers called these unproductive lands "waste land," a term that did not exist in the Indigenous imagination (Pelzer 1978, 71).[3] Villages lost their religious, political, and ecological functions when the land was constructed primarily for economic pursuits. In Batak Indigenous wisdom,[4] the land is never wasted. Human absence on land does not mean wasting the land. The land for the Batak people is sacred, gifted by God.[5]

Each type of land performs various functionalities that are opposed to capitalistic views of land productivity. Bungaran Simanjuntak, a Batak sociologist, identifies different types and functions of land, such as *tano tarulang* (untouched land), *tano na niulang* (intentionally abandoned land for planting transition time), *harangan/tombak* (forest), *hauma* (rice field), *pargadongan* (nonrice field), *tano parhutaan* (residential land/village), *jalangan/jampalan* (farming areas with pasture), and *parmualan* (wetlands for water).[6] Some lands left empty or even untouched were meant for preservation. Moreover, deep *harangan* was often untouched as a mystery space, believed to be a space for the divine's immanent presence, comparable to the Jewish belief in the mountains. *Tano na niulang* represents the necessary time for the land to heal and regenerate its fertility called "*boraspati ni tano*." *Boraspati ni tano* is

---

3. Decree No. 4 of 27 January 1877 and the 1878's decree were the first two model contracts that reflected the Western legal concepts exercised in stipulating the land concessions.

4. Bungaran Antonius Simanjuntak, *Arti dan Fungsi Tanah Bagi Masyarakat Batak Toba, Karo, Simalungun* (Edisi Pembaruan), (Jakarta: Yayasan Pustaka Obor Indonesia, 2015), 21–4.

5. A short description of how the earth or land began according to the Batak mythology may be found in Sibeth, 1991, 65. Four versions of creation Batak mythology can be found in Siagian 2016, 233–73.

6. Simanjuntak, *Arti dan Fungsi Tanah Bagi Musyarakat*, 21–4. I have also discussed the Batak theology of land at length in Hesron H. Sihombing, "The Batak-Christian Theology of Land: Towards a Postcolonial Comparative Theology," *CrossCurrents* 73, no. 1 (2023): 42–63, https://doi.org/10.1353/cro.2023.0003.

symbolized by the brown skink (*Eutropis multifasciata*) and also associated with breasts as symbols of new life, fertility, and prosperity. Therefore, the Batak conception of the land illustrates things beyond economic life, reflecting the cultural, spiritual, ecological, and women's roles.

During the Dutch colonization era, what separated the Toba Batak's experience from the rest of East Sumatra and other Batak areas was that no plantations had developed in the Toba Batak areas. This is due to their opposition to agrarian law and their rejection of the "waste land" concept of their Indigenous land. They realized it would be disastrous for their land to be let into the plantations' possessions. With the help of the RMG missionaries, the Batak Christians wrote resolutions and petitions to reject the granting of concessions and long leases (Pelzer 1978, 91). The missionaries did this ultimately out of worry about the potential import of Muslim Javanese workers to the region if the plantations went through. The Toba Batak's protests, nonetheless, were based on *adat* (traditional custom) claims that all lands were connected to the *marga* or clans. Traditionally, land ownership was established when one clan settled a village in a formerly unoccupied place. Ownership became communal, albeit exclusively attached to one particular clan. In this way, as Paul Pedersen notes, founding a new village was less about gaining material wealth than improving social prestige (Pedersen 1970, 34). However, I argue that people's attachment to a village was more rooted in its function as a social organization in which people connected to a specific marga formed communal and ecological relationships among themselves and nature. The Batak Christians used this cultural understanding of land as bound to a community's identity to argue that permission for land use had to be acquired from the marga representatives (Pelzer 1978, 91), none of whom would allow any land to fall into planters' hands.

However, like other groups, the Toba Batak suffered from high taxation levied by the Dutch colonizers of 6 Rupiah (1 Rupiah = 36 liters (about 9.51 gal of rice), equivalent to 216 liters (about 57.06 gal) of unhusked rice.[7] This high taxation forced the Batak people to produce

---

7. Detailed information on the taxation especially in the Samosir island area may be found in Sherman, 2020.

more rice, changing their cultural perspective and worldview of cultivating enough, respecting the soil, and connecting with nature. Thus, when the colonizers failed to acquire the land, they devised taxation to break the Indigenous culture's practices of land cultivation. Maarten Manse, a Dutch colonial historian, highlights how taxation around the world, including in Indonesia, can be seen as "an exercise in Foucauldian governance and state-building to map societies, instill new forms of behavior, and standardize, discipline, and 'civilize' subject populations" (Manse 2022, 421). In different parts of colonial Indonesia, high taxation was levied to "[assess] and [repair] hostile attitudes toward the Dutch" and to "acquire information, implement governance, and change social realities" (422). Taxes were purposefully made higher so the local people would not spend their money on idle pursuits or even to organize raids (422). For food colonialism to function, it had to destroy the Indigenous culture of food resources and transform or "docilize" the objects (in this case, the land, rice, and people) at the center of Indigenous culture so they would align with the insidious purpose of colonial capitalism.

The plantation economy spread rapidly in the East Sumatra region, especially the Karo and Simalungun areas, while the locals gradually lost their land rights. Kozok states that by 1938, European plantation owners had occupied one-third of the Simalungun area and used it for plantations (Kozok 1991, 35). The plantations represent the industrial capitalist economy, which planted rubber, palm oil, cocoa, tea, tobacco, coconut, nutmeg, sugar, coffee, indigo, and other products for export in various East Sumatra areas. The local Simalungunese refused to work in the plantations because the work required prolonged and intensive work hours. To work on the plantations, the Dutch colonial government brought in Malay Chinese and Javanese "coolies," who by 1921 had reached a total of forty-four thousand people, some settled in new villages. The wage policy of the planters was to pay each worker depending on the quality and quantity of the product (Pelzer 1978, 35).

This enormous growth of population required more food production. Karl Pelzer notes that the colonial government would have to produce twice as much rice as the annual production of 180,000 tons. This condition forced them to require plantations to release lands for food production

(119). A report indicates that, in 1909, around 68,764 tons of rice, of which four-sevenths came from Rangoon, was imported to fill the need gaps in East Sumatra.[8] The colonial administration then migrated the Toba Batak people to these plantation areas, promising new land and settlement if they produced rice and provided a sound irrigation system for paddy-field cultivation. It even provided a system of credit known as "Tobaneesche Landbouwbank" for agricultural loans. Kozok records that around twenty-five thousand Toba and Mandailing people migrated to the Simalungun areas from 1907 to 1921 (Kozok 1991, 35–36). Clark Cunningham, an American anthropologist working on Indonesia and Thailand, reports that the colonial government allocated the Toba settlers one hectare (2.47 acres) of wetland per family, or one-half hectare for bachelors. They were prohibited from selling or transferring the land without the permission of the colonial government and Simalungunese kings, who acquired the land taxes (Cunningham 1958, 86).

German missionaries also supported this massive migration to facilitate the evangelization of the Simalungun people (Asnewastri 2018, 16–17). The Simalungun became a minority and owned the least of their own lands. In addition, well-educated migrants from Tapanuli, one of the Toba Batak areas, also flooded the plantation areas. The missionaries built schools centered around Western education to teach the Toba Batak people. Many of them were well educated from these elementary schools and later discovered that education could play a prominent role in elevating their economic and social status. With this comparably high-level education, they could find higher positions with better wages at the plantation areas and foreign companies (Purba and Purba 1997, 65–66).[9] They

---

8. "No. 4925 Annual Series. Diplomatic and Consular Reports, Netherlands, Report for the Year 1911 on the Trade and Commerce, &c., of Java, Sumatra, &c, Edited at the Foreign Office and the Board of Trade. Reference to Previous Report, Annual Series No. 4670.," Diplomatic and Consular Reports (London: His Majesty's Stationery Office, 1912), https://parlipapers-proquest-com.du.idm.oclc.org/parlipapers/result/pqpdocumentview?accountid=14608&groupid=95822&pgId=de856e89-f132-4c9e-bcdb-dedf5dc30b66&rsId=18E42B3F7AA#59, 36.

9. The Purbas indicate that the number of schools built by the RMG missionaries in Tapanuli (one of the Toba Batak areas) surpassed the ones built by the colonial govern-

worked as office workers in the plantations. When they migrated to the cities, they worked as clerks in private companies or government services (Cunningham 1958, 87).

Cunningham states that from 1915 to 1930, the colonial government built around 35,540 acres of wet-rice land in Sidamanik and Tanah Jawa of the Simalungun areas. The migration and settlement of the Toba Batak people contributed to this development. With this population increase of the Toba Batak people and the development of the wet rice land, the Simalungunese lost the space for alternative cultivation and withdrew to the fringe areas of the new rice fields or highland regions. As minorities, they could not accept living together with the Toba Batak, whom they thought to be aggressive (Cunningham 1958, 85). Cunningham reports that there were 48,571 Toba Bataks in Simalungun and 17,966 in Asahan in 1930.

The movement of the Toba Batak was measured and limited according to the plantations' needs. Just a few Toba Bataks were allowed to migrate to other regions. Cunningham records that in Langkat, there were only 411 Toba Bataks compared to 217,857 Indonesians in total in the same year. In Deli Serdang, there were 2,472 Toba Bataks compared to 431,599 Indonesians. Both areas were centers of plantations (Cunningham 1958, 86), but were indirectly ruled by the colonial government. In Simalungun, colonial rule was arranged directly, making the concession areas the designated destinations of the Dutch-facilitated Toba Batak migration. Besides, in the Deli Serdang, Langkat, Batu Bara, and Asahan areas, the sultans and most of society had converted to Islam. They worked closely with the Western-owned plantations and the Dutch colonizers. The sultans would not welcome the Toba Batak to migrate to their areas. The Toba Batak had an "unpleasant and even perilous experience" in these regions, as they were not allowed to build churches. The Muslim coastal people socially alienated them as traditional rumors still held them to be pagans and cannibals (Cunningham 1958, 87–88).

This reality tells us that in the massive production of food, the food colonization system organized food resources. But even more, the system

---

ment. In 1936 alone, the mission body owned 585 schools with 43,184 students compared to 13,635 students in 159 government-owned schools.

utilized some "docilized" Indigenous people to meet its production goals through migration. The Toba Batak migration was only possible when the Toba Batak culture was first destroyed and life in their traditional land was made harder due to high Dutch-levied taxation. By invoking a capitalistic mentality of rapid upward economic mobility, Western education and systematic migration became tools to accelerate the process of food colonization. Western education that did not honor Indigenous traditions contributed heavily to the loss of Indigenous culture of food and the imposition of capitalistic ways of life. It was only when Indigenous people were deprived of their cultural wisdom that they could be effectively included in the capitalistic modes of production. The inclusion of Indigenous people in the capitalistic economy marked the intricate relationships between colonialism, Western education, capitalism, and migration. This was when the Toba Batak people started to embrace their newly constructed identity as *bangso pangaranto* (settled foreigners). Their guiding principle turned to *hamajuon* (advancement), which mainly materialized into social prestige (*hasangapon*) and material wealth (*hamoraon*) (Purba and Purba 1997, 70–71; Keuning 1958, 14).

In addition to the Toba Batak, the Minang, Angkola, and Mandailing Batak people, mostly Muslims, flocked to the near-coastal areas of East Sumatra. Unlike the Toba Batak, they were more readily accepted in these areas because most of society had converted to Islam. The planters employed them as clerks, surveyors, mechanics, and in other minor positions (Pelzer 1978, 60). The structure of society was transformed so that the original landowners were set against marginalized workers from different ethnic and religious backgrounds.

RICE AND *MARSIADAPARI* IN BATAK CULTURE

For the Batak people, rice was never a product for the market. As part of collective work called *marsiadapari*, planting and harvesting rice embodies the importance of community. The village community planted rice to harvest annually to provide enough for the whole village and save some portions for the dry season or emergencies. However, rice did not just serve as the staple food but had theological and cultural meanings. Rice is also used as "*boras si pir ni tondi*" (rice as the spirit amplifier). The Batak people believe that when accompanied by prayers, rice can strengthen the human soul or spirit, just like a grain of rice is firm. According to Resmi Hutasoit, Izak M. Lattu, and Ebenhaizer I Nuban Timo, besides the firm texture of the rice grain, there are three reasons rice is symbolized as the spirit amplifier. First, it fulfills human bodily needs. Second, since people of any social status can have rice, it fosters a sense of social equality. Third, when rice is spread to touch human bodies, it does not hurt them (2020, 18). This may seem odd in the Western imagination, but in the Bataks' worldview, the spirit and body are different but inseparable domains, similar to the view of relations between the individual and the community. The fulfillment of bodily needs is directly linked to spiritual fulfillment, and the satisfaction of one's spirit extensively entails community flourishing.

In special events, such as entering a new house, a wedding, or escaping danger, *boras si pir ni tondi*, which is uncooked, is scattered on the head of the recipient along with words of poem and prayers, "*Mardangka ma baringin, di mual Pulo Batu; Horas tondi madingin, pir tondi matogu*" which means "may your soul find peace and strength."[10] Different prayers are spoken depending on the occasion. When a family enters a new house, the rice is spread in different corners of the house with the hope that the family may have strong spirits when inhabiting it (Hutasoit et al. 2020, 186). Someone who escapes danger receives *boras si pir ni tondi* to bring their spirit to their body, as it is believed that the endangerment has separated one's spirit from the body, leading to the person's absentmindedness, trauma, or confusion. By doing this, the person can become a complete human being and regain the strength to face life again.

Batak people also serve rice in its flour form. Rice flour, grated coconut, sugar, and salt are mixed and pressed together to make uncooked rice flour cakes called "*itak gurgur*." As its name—the boiling rice flour—suggests, people eat *itak gurgur* to "heat up" the feckless spirit. The *itak gurgur* tradition of blessing also reaches beyond humans. *Itak gurgur*, represented

10. Felix Tani, "Bagi Orang Batak, Beras Bukan Sekadar Makanan Pokok," *Kompasiana* (blog), accessed August 28, 2023, https://www.kompasiana.com/mtf3lix5tr/5c82166faeebe13beb3ae952/bagi-orang-batak-beras-bukan-sekadar-makanan-pokok?page=all#section2.

by lime juice, is splashed on rice plants when they reach the generative phase. The Batak believe the rice plants already possess their souls or spirits in this phase. By splashing the itak gurgur with prayers, the farmers encourage the rice plants to grow healthy to produce good crops.[11] Anicetus Sinaga states that the actual *itak*, when offered to the gods along with the cooked rice, symbolizes the fertility of rice fields and cattle. Prayers are lifted during the offering rites with the hope for fertile soils and rain (2014, 136–37).

Rice also mediates human relationships. By serving and eating *indahan na las* (the warm rice) together, the warmth and joy of the heart are shared in the community. After eating rice, conversations about disputes and reconciliation, requests and inheritance, and others may proceed. Eating is a sacred action. Even a thief cannot be caught while eating. Rice contains meaning (*indahan na marlapatan*) because eating rice is preceded by calling the intention of serving the food and words of blessing (Sinaga 2014, 194–95). For Batak people, food, especially rice, serves symbolic, sacred, and pastoral functions. Rice's production and consumption symbolize the strength of the soul, love and care in the community, and human collective relationship with the divine. Rice must be respected because it possesses a soul and can strengthen human souls. To waste even just one grain of rice means disrespecting God, God's blessings, the rice, nature, and farmers.

This culture started to change when the colonial administration introduced the market economy. Colonizers built transportation systems using forced labor. With the new transportation system, the Europeans created vegetable plantations for crops like potatoes and cabbages in the Karo plateau, and the products could reach Medan quickly to be exported to Penang (Malaysia) and Singapore. The Batak people, including the non-Toba ones, started shifting their economy from a subsistence to a market economy. Different reasons caused this. Some Batak were driven by the burden of meeting the high taxation that boosted productivity; some saw this as an opportunity for economic growth and imitated the cultivation methods of the plantations. They started to grow produce solely for market purposes, such as vegetables, fruit, coffee, and cloves, where Singapore and Malaysia

11. Tani, "Bagi Orang Batak."

served as the most projected markets. The trade was mediated by Chinese dealers who often provided credit to local farmers (Kozok 1991, 37).

The Simalungunese began to grow vegetables for the market, seeking to cover high taxation. They also grew coffee for the market like the Mandailing people did. In Toba land in Tapanuli, the Toba Batak shifted towards growing rubber for export (Kozok 1991, 35–36). In Toba Batak's homeland, rice became an industrial commodity for market purposes. In addition to being forced by Dutch-imposed high taxation to produce more rice, the Toba Batak people also sold rice to meet the increasing demands of the European plantation population outside the Toba area. The primary focus of production became profit. These exclusively marketed products boosted the use of artificial fertilizers and pesticides, leaving the fallow periods to create two or three harvest times annually. Planting rice loses its communal sense as profit becomes the ultimate purpose. This condition led to ecological destruction, such as massive deforestation, soil damage, and erosion.

Food colonialism changed the cultural value of rice. Furthermore, it changed the way rice is produced. The Toba Batak people cultivated rice through the communal practice called "*marsiadapari*," a tradition that rarely appears today. The word "*marsiadapari*" literally means "taking or picking up other people's working day for several days" (Sibarani 2018, 49). It is a tradition in which a group of five to six people in a village work together to plant and harvest the rice field without a wage. They take turns working on the group members' rice fields in the spirit of unity and love (Siahaan et al. 2022, 1031), working alternately from one field to the next until every member's rice field is worked. Manat Siahaan et al. portray *marsiadapari* as a practice of reciprocal togetherness that is not limited to economic activities. By lending our hands to help others in the group, the others will do the same for us. By working on our neighbors' rice fields, they will, in turn, work on our rice fields. In this practice, the Batak proverb says, "*si solisoli do uhum, siadapari gogo*," meaning "if you give, you will be given" (1031). The literal meaning of the proverb is "reciprocity is law, helping each other is strength."

Male members of the community usually do more physical work, such as hoeing and plowing, and female members plant the rice. The task can be finished early as everyone maintains their work pace with the spirit of laboring together. The essential features of this practice lie in the principles of equality, friendship, and compatibility. The members share the work equally with a similar workload to complete. The groups are formed impermanently and are usually dissolved at the end of a particular task. Leadership is not necessary, although occasionally, the owner of a specific rice field might provide some advice and direction. A person who drops out in the middle of the work must find someone from their family to substitute for them. Cunningham argues that this agricultural practice "gives greater pleasure to the workers, and therein lies its profit" (Cunningham 1958, 54).

Food colonialism that individualizes and commodifies rice diminishes the practice of *marsiadapari* because it does not correspond with the spirit of capitalism. The postcolonial Indonesian government recently launched a "food estate" program whereby forests were cleared for large-scale food production, including rice, cassava, and potatoes. One of the food estate sites is in Batak land. Intended to create national food sustainability, the project has failed due to a lack of proper planning, leaving the plantations abandoned and awaiting ecological destruction, which affects the surrounding local communities. Some environmental and Indigenous activists have expressed their criticism of this program as it has contributed to local farmers' crop failure, land destruction, agrarian conflict, the loss of forest areas, and Indigenous peoples' devastation of their traditional economic sources (KSPPM, 2021).[12] Moreover, the project does not promote the community's involvement in the practice of marsiadapari.

Colonialism changed the meaning of rice to become merely "productive food" for the sake of the market and capitalistic economy. By imposing a colonial understanding of food, colonial power maintains its economic dominance and enables the colonizers to sustain its authoritative reach at

12. This book is an anthology of responses from the Batak activists and scholars on food estate. They criticize food estate and corporate-based food production. These authors suggest that food or farmer sovereignty should be the solution to achieve food security, whereby the locals and Indigenous communities should have self-determination to decide on their food policy and production.

the cultural, religious, and political levels. The market economy has replaced the subsistence and community-based economy, negatively affecting how the Batak people view the economy, land, food, and community. Food is a powerful tool within and for colonization.

Revitalizing *marsiadapari* practice in the Batak community can become the source of resistance against food colonialism. This practice's principles extend beyond agricultural activities to encompass mutual cooperation, community building and flourishing, and human connectedness with nature. These essential principles oppose the conventions of rapid and massive crop production, abuse of land, and cheap labor relations. This practice teaches the Batak people to form strong and needed coalitions and unity for their food and communal sovereignty. In this collective practice, they learn to honor the rice fields, nature, and community and to reinvent rice's cultural and theological meanings.

SECTION VI

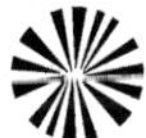

OCEANIA

16

They Took Our Fish and Sold Us Their Tin Fish (Canned Fish)!

'Ikani Fakasi'i'eiki

Pacific Island peoples are known for their hospitality, friendliness, and unique celebrations called luau. They love to come together to eat and talk as relatives and in communities. Cooking and eating are presented in celebratory and communal ways, with the bulk of the food harvested, collected, and prepared using traditional cooking practices such as wrapping the food to be cooked in *lu* (leaves) and then arranging the layers of the food in *umu* (underground ovens). Communities typically spend much time over the course of days or months preparing for these gatherings, making sure the food from the land and the sea is ready at just the right time.

Food culture is key in sustaining the people over generations. Food culture was and still is a source of connection, a way of passing knowledges from one generation to another, a source of life for the people. In the islands, calendars and knowledge were passed on in a sharing of the wisdom of known growing seasons and their connection to the lunar cycles. These instructions sometimes included elaborate rituals to stimulate memory of when to plant and when to harvest, when to feast and when to fast.

Fresh food from the sea and land was readily available to anyone who had the knowledge of how to gather food, farm, and fish. These knowledges were, for the most part, cut off when colonial powers began to engage with the islanders. As a result of external influences, food culture has become a point of division that has undermined family ties. That communal food culture was replaced with a competitive commodified food culture that prioritizes profit over community, land, sea and harvesting rights, which in turn, has become a source of disease and death. In this chapter, I will discuss the historical impact of colonialism on people's health, and in particular their lifestyle and nutrition, and its reverberations in the Pacific Islands today. I will explore how colonialism has affected these small islands' way of life and their nutrition and health, which has led to them being dependent upon and controlled by outside governments and companies.

COLONIALISM IN THE PACIFIC ISLANDS

Colonialism occurs when a dominant power establishes control over Indigenous people with the purpose of exploitation and expansion. Colonialism in the Pacific came in two different forms. The first form of colonialism was a result of interisland and panoceanic navigation by explorers from other islands. Oral history describes that Tonga built and expanded its empire throughout Oceania around the period of 1200 to 1500 CE. Islands from the other parts of Oceania were subjected to the *Tu'i Tonga* (king), who brought *'inasi* (tribute), including fruits of the land, crafts, mats, and other gifts. As a result, many of the fine imports from these distant islands were brought and kept as treasures in the islands of Tonga. The tributes that were offered led to intermarriage between ethnic groups, especially between the children of chiefs from Samoa, Fiji, and Tonga. The decline of the Tongan empire led to Samoan and other islands expelling the Tongans. These islands were then able to rule their own islands or develop their own systems of ruling that fit each island's contexts.

The second phase of colonization came to the Pacific Islands between the sixteenth and eighteenth centuries. By the end of the twentieth century, almost all of the islands except Tonga had been colonized by either the American, European, or Asian powers. The Europeans, Americans, and Asians viewed these small island countries as empty places that needed to be governed and civilized. Their small size, lack of military resources, isolation, and self-contained rule made them ideal places to take over and control. The bigger countries with more power and resources not only overwhelmed these small islands easily, but simply enveloped them without initially using military force or warfare, although at other times war became another mechanism to usurp power.

Political colonization in the Pacific has always gone hand in hand with the expansion of Christianity and international trade. Christian missionaries viewed the islanders as heathen savages who needed to be civilized and converted to the new religion. Some missionaries referred to this effort as helping the native peoples to be "cleansed from all sin" and impurity (Chidester 2001, 472). Their imposition of this new religion and Western customs on islanders impacted all areas of life: spirituality, culture, education, and family. Indigenous culture was referred to as sinful and unclean, while the Western way of life was considered to be good, clean, and pure. One scholar referred to the coming of European colonization, which included political, military, and religious replacements, as "set from darkness to light" (Yannick 2011, 461–72).

The missionaries paved the way for foreign governments to move into these small islands to take possession of and gain control over all aspects of society. The heavy involvement of these outside powers together with internal political instability made it easier for the conquerors to occupy the islands. Colonizers believed that these island countries needed law and order, which meant the Western forms of law and constitution, but they ignored the fact that these islands countries had been self-governed for many generations. These new forms of law and order were meant to control and dominate the native people on their own lands, including banning many native ways of doing things. The missionaries and the Westerners lack of knowledge of the Indigenous lifestyle and way of doing things led them to quickly deny, negate, or have disdain for Indigenous knowledges. In doing so, from a missionary perspective, both Indigenous knowledges and local healers and their medicine were either discredited, devalued, or condemned as "evil." Fer Yannick describes the encounter between Christianity and the local beliefs that generated manifestations of religious intolerance, "witch-hunting being the most spectacular" (2011,

461). This ideology not only forced them to practice the religion of the colonizers, but also expanded to coerce them to abhor all aspects of their life, including religious, social, economic, educational, cultural, and other.

In addition to replacing Indigenous religion and government, foreign trade was established, and other forms of control followed suit. In 1857, J. C. Godeffroy and Son launched in Apia, becoming the biggest trading company in the Islands (Bollard 1981, 3). This merchant venture firm played a major role in colonial struggle and colonial domination in the Pacific both in Tonga and Samoa. They also were the lead in introducing a "series of economic innovation in the South Pacific, setting pattern of commercial development in the 19th and early 20th centuries" (Bollard 1981, 3).

The First World War had a great impact on these small island countries. Australia took over New Guinea, later naming it Papua New Guinea. New Zealand took over the islands of Samoa, previously controlled by Germany. Japan inserted itself as a new superpower, taking possession of the Marshall Islands, Palau, and the Mariana Islands. The changing of external powers in the islands continued to bring tension to these small island nations. At the same time, conflict between the superpowers added another layer of fear for islanders. The Great Depression of the 1930s affected all the islands, leading to the fluctuation of the market for products such as copra, banana, sugar, and other foods. This period brought new diseases, such as malaria and epidemics. These foreign diseases were unfamiliar to Indigenous healers. By that time, most Indigenous healers and their native medicines had already been banned or marginalized as a resulted of colonization. So, the islanders did not have the resources to cure those foreign sicknesses. However, at that time, they began to rely on the colonial doctors for medical cures, which gave more power to the colonial authorities.[1]

---

1. Keily Leina'ala Kawakami, Shelly Muneoka, Rachel Burrage, Leslie Tanoue, Kilohana Haitsuka and Kathryn Braun, "The Lives of Native Hawaiian Elders and Their Experiences with Healthcare: A Qualitative Analysis," Front Public Health, 2022; 10:787215, doi: 10.3389/fpubh.2022.797215., Feb 22, 2022. Also, refer to the study of Mai Misaki, *"Rā'au mā'ohi*: the Efficacy and Resurgence of Traditional Herbal Medicine in French Polynesia," *Open Edition Journals*, p.245-258, https://doi.org/10.400/jso.13134., 2021.

The Second World War directly affected these island countries in every aspect. They continued to be exposed to European, American, and Japanese influences, which over time became more extensive. The end of the war led to a major reshuffling of colonial powers. By the mid-twentieth century, almost all the islands had been colonized at one point or another. While some islands gained their independence, others continued under colonial rule, with some colonial powers beginning to allow Indigenous leaders to be a part of their colonial governments. Although some of these islands began to obtain their independence, the influence of the colonial powers continued to be strong, extending that influence to the independent governments. For example, France continued to hold onto Tahiti and the United States held Hawaii. By the mid-twentieth century, China became another major foreign power to have more presence in the Pacific. All these foreign powers still maintain their heavy influence on trade, economic and political life, including nutrition and lifestyle. The islands were exposed to more foreign ways of life and living, such as European, American, and Asian, forcing islanders to live as foreigners in their own lands.

FOOD AND DISEASE IN THE PACIFIC

The process of colonization, including the imposition of international food trade methods and foreign diets, had a negative impact on the life and health of islanders (Hughes and Lawrence 2005, 298–306). When they first arrived to these islands, some scholars described the people as healthy and muscular, referring to "primitives affluence" (Fisk 1966, 23). For example, in the journal of Captain James Cook, written throughout his travels across the Pacific, he described the healthy life and healthy diet of the people in the islands, including Tonga, the Cook Islands, Tahiti, and others (Hughes 2003, 7). This healthy life was disrupted by contact with the Europeans and their colonial rule. Although these small island nations now seemed to be free from political colonial powers as independent nations, the colonial imprint has been embedded deeply in these island countries, especially in the realm of food culture and food resources as part of their nutrition, education, and economy, as well as their social and religious beliefs.

Food culture was usurped, and food was expected to be prepared according to colonial methods and diets. Anthropologists Amy K.

McLennan and Stanley J. Ulijaszek describe how Westerners taught islanders "proper" food habits as part of their attempt to civilize them (McLennan and Ulijaszek 2015, 1499–505). The colonizers educated the native people about the proper "colonized" ways to make food and eat. All instructions were formulated according to colonial ways and lifestyles. McLennan and Ulijaszek describe how a wife of one of the missionaries in Nauru proudly shared that she was able to convince the native people of Nauru that eating raw fish, among other native food practices, was not good (McLennan and Ulijaszek 2015, 1499–505). In addition, part of her mission to civilize islanders was to teach them proper nutrition and cooking, which meant Western nutritional customs. That led to many islanders losing their authentic connection with traditional food growing and preparation skills and their becoming more dependent on imported unhealthy food.[2] In addition, they started adding foreign food to their diet. Island communities' food preparation was originally a communal activity; but when colonial food preparation practices were becoming the norm, separation into individual households became more accepted. Christian missionaries were responsible for imposing onto these islanders' formal education and "proper" ways of life. They were not only taught this through proper formal education, but these ways were also persistently forced through informal daily interactions.

The Western way of life was not only regarded as the better way but also became the considered norm. The islanders were forced to regard native foods as inferior, which led them to be persuaded against eating local foods or to eliminate them from their diets altogether. The new ways of life carried with them new demands, including new forms of nutrients and food systems. The new things, including new diseases that they brought to these islands, were not something that Indigenous healers nor medicine were accustomed to curing. In many circumstances these new diseases caused much death for the Indigenous populations. More than 70 percent of deaths across the Pacific region are caused by

---

2. McLennan and Ulijazek 2015, 1499–1505., Also refer to Jessica Ruikka, "The Western diet's impact on the health of Pacific Islands," College of Arts & Science Senior Honor Thesis Paper 99, hhttp://doi.org/10.18297/honors/99, 2016.

noncommunicable diseases (NCD's), many of which can be traced back to unhealthy diets and poor nutrition.[3] According to the World Health Organization (WHO), unhealthy diet and poor nutrition are the leading contributors to global disease, including obesity and other NCD's (Hughes and Lawrence 2005, 298). Some island countries in the South Pacific rank among the most obese countries in the world.[4] This is largely attributable to the high level of unhealthy Western processed and cast-off food, including mutton flaps, turkey tails, and other canned food imported to the islands and sold as staple parts of daily diet.

In the Pacific, the most sought-after cuts of meat now include cuts that are considered off limits to the palates of citizens of colonial powers. At Thanksgiving, one of the most celebrated holidays in United States, more than 80 percent of US families enjoy turkey for dinner.[5] However, turkey tails, the fattiest part of the turkey, are never recognized as part of the dinner for US families. Beginning in the 1950s, instead of throwing out turkey and chicken tails, the global food industry saw an opportunity for additional profit and targeted Pacific Island consumers, primarily the market in Samoa.[6] That unhealthy cut of meat later become one of the more common foods in Samoa, accepted as part of the main dish in their

---

3. The World Bank Group, "Pacific Island: Non-Commutable Disease Roadmap," July 12, 2014, https://www.worldbank.org/en/news/feature/2014/07/11/pacific-islands-non-communicable-disease-roadmap.

4. World Bank Group, "Pacific Island." See also the recent study by the WHO, Western Pacific, "Study finds Pacific account for 9 of the 10 most obese countries in the world," March 4, 2024, https://www.who.int/westernpacific/about/how-we-work/pacific-support/news/detail/04-03-2024-study-finds-pacific-accounts-for-9-of-the-10-most-obese-countries-in-the-world#:~:text=©-,Study%20finds%20Pacific%20accounts%20for%209%20of%20the,obese%20countries%20in%20the%20world&text=New%20analysis%20published%20in%20the,men%20aged%2020%20and%20above,.

5. Michael Carolan, "The strange story of turkey tails speaks volumes about our globalized food system," *The Conversation*, November 12, 2017, https://theconversation.com/the-strange-story-of-turkey-tails-speaks-volumes-about-our-globalized-food-system-86035. The same article was republished in Atlas Obscura as "How Turkey Tails Became a National Dish in Samoa," November 15, 2021, https://www.atlasobscura.com/articles/turkey-tails.

6. Carolan, "The strange story of turkey tails."

meals. New Zealand and Australian food companies also began exporting to the Pacific their meat cuts that were unacceptable to their other consumers, such as fatty mutton flaps, beef, and canned meat.[7] Also, unwanted pork meat was turned into Spam to provide food for US soldiers, which later became the most popular food in many islands in the Pacific, especially the Micronesian islands. Hughes and Lawrence refer to this as food "dumping" (Hughes and Lawrence 2005, 299). They also mention how other scholars called this toxic colonial food system "dietary colonialism," "Coca-colonialism," and "dietary genocide."

The contact of the island nations with Europeans, Americans, and Asians brought to these small islands new ways of life, including new forms of disease, but also created a culture of competition and rivalry that valued money over community and relationships. This communal life where resources are shared has been discouraged and abandoned. As these island nations entered into transnational free trade agreements, their experience has been one of losing their voice at the decision-making table. The trade agreements stipulated that local "exotic" food could be harvested and exported for consumption abroad for high profits of food corporations.[8] In practice, when local food is exported and controlled by outsiders, that means that local resources are either no longer available for local communities or too expensive compared with imported food. This leads to increased dependency on unhealthy imported products. When this transnational trade was formed, these small islands countries had no choice but to be part of these trade partnerships. They are powerless, with no voice in the trade agreement; therefore, they just have to go along. For

7. Carolan, "The strange story of turkey tails." See also Svati Kristen Narula, "Thanks for mutton, New Zealand: Your fatty meat products are making Tonga obese," *Quartz*, January 20, 2016, https://qz.com/597669/thanks-for-the-mutton-new-zealand-your-fatty-meat-products-are-making-tonga-obese.

8. T. D. Brewer, N. L. Andrew, D. Abbott, R. Detenamo, E. N. Faaola, P. V. Gounder, N. Lal, K. Lui, A. Ravuvu, D. Sapalojang, M. K. Sharp, R. J. Sulu, S. Suvulo, J. M. M. M. Tamate, A. M. Thow, A. T. Wells, "The role of trade in Pacific food security and nutrition," in *Global Food Security*, 36, 100670 (March 2023), https://doi.org/10.1016/j.gfs.2022.100670.

example, Samoa banned the import of turkey tails in 2007.[9] However, under World Trade Organization rules, countries and territories generally cannot ban the import of any commodities unless they prove that there are public health reasons for doing so. So, to join the WTO, Samoa had to lift its ban on turkey tails in 2013.[10]

These trade agreements played a major role in shaping the national food environment and the nutritional quality of the food supply sent to the Pacific Islands.[11] The participation of Pacific Island nations in global free trade agreements, which affect local government decisions, increased the penetration of food and beverages by global corporations through swift urbanization, which has expanded the access of the people to processed food even in the most remote areas in the islands. Rapid Westernization of these islands has made processed food more appealing, available, and accessible to island populations, which has simultaneously resulted in more widespread health impacts, such as NCDs.

Since Pacific Islanders love group feasting and culture of celebration, foreign food industries and business owners take advantage of it. Churches, instead of speaking against the unhealthiness of these foods that people put on feast tables, take advantage of the situation to attract people as an opportunity to raise funds for the church.

In response to the dietary concerns related to the spread of NCDs, some Pacific Islands have changed the policy of liberal trade and the process of external companies and products penetrating the food market and the food environment, especially the processes that promote cheap

---

9. Anne Marie Thow, Boyd Swinburn, Stephen Colagiuri, Mere Diligolevu, Christine Quested, Paula Vivili, and Stephen Leeder, "Trade and food policy: Case studies from three Pacific Island countries," Food Policy, *Elsevier*, 35,6 (December 2010), 556–64.

10. Anna Marie Thow, Erica Reeve, Take Naseri, Tim Martyn, and Caroline Bollars, "Food supply, nutrition and trade policy: reversal of an important ban on turkey tails," Bulletin World Health Organization 95,10 (October 1, 2017), 723–25, published online Aug 23, doi. 10.2471/BLT.17.192468; See also Carolan, "The strange story of turkey tails."

11. A. M. Thow et al., "Food trade among Pacific Island countries and territories: implications for food security and nutrition," *Global Health* 18, 104 (December 14, 2022), https://doi.org/10.1186/s12992-022-00891-9.

and convenient processed foods that are high in salt, sugar, and fat.[12] However, in trying to create policies to combat that issue, the policy makers have been faced with strong opposition from food and beverage companies, which attempt to overturn these policies and pressure island governments to minimize their moratorium on imported food policies in trade.[13] Another effort to address the issue of a moratorium on importing processed food to these island nations has been to increase the promotion of sustainable agricultural practices by reintroducing organic farming. For example, in August 2023, Tonga marked a significant step towards attaining sustainable agricultural practices and fostering a healthier nutrition lifestyle by publicizing that they successfully launched two organic farms. These two farms are part of the project called Pacific Organic Learning Farms Network (POLFN).[14] This attempt to enter into organic farming embraces the idea to farm without using chemicals. However, that was their statement instead of saying that this kind of farming will return the process to native or Indigenous ways of farming, because that was how our ancestors and elders did their farming and growing food.

THE FISHERY TREATY BETWEEN THE UNITED STATES AND THE PACIFIC ISLANDS

The Pacific Ocean is home to the largest tuna population on Earth. Tuna fisheries are vital for the life of these small islands in the Pacific. They support "food security" and the economies of the Pacific Island countries. The South Pacific Tuna Treaty was implemented between the United States and sixteen Pacific Island countries in 1988 and was extended in 1993,

---

12. Emilee Walby, Amanda C. Jones, Moira Smith, Elisiva Na'ati, Wendy Snowdon, and Andrea M Teng, "Food Tax Policies in Pacific Island Countries and Territories: Systematic Policy Review." NIH National Library of Medicine, Public Health Nutrition 2024; 27(1):e20, doi:10.1017/S1368980023002914.

13. Erica Reeve, Prabhat Lamichhane, Briar McKenzie, Gade Waqa, Jacqui Webster, Wendy Snowdon, and Colin Bell, "The tide of dietary risks for noncommunicable diseases in Pacific Islands: an analysis of population NCD surveys," *BMC Public Health* 22 (August 10, 2022), 1521, https://doi.org/10.1186/s12889-022-13808-3.

14. Newsdesk, "Tonga launches organic learning farms to transform food system," August 9, 2023, https://talanoaotonga.to/tonga-launches-organic-learning-farms-to-transform-food-system/.

2002, and again in 2022.[15] The South Pacific Tuna Treaty allows US fishing vessels to freely fish for tuna in the exclusive economic zones of the treaty parties without interruption. In return, the United States agreed to provide economic assistance to the Pacific Island nations, which seemed to offer help to these islands, but in the end the United States benefitted more than the Pacific Islands. In 2021, about sixteen US fishing vessels were allocated to fish around the area.[16] Also, longline fishing is the main tool used for tuna fishing by most of the fishing vessels currently in the Pacific from China, Taiwan, or other outside countries registered in one of the islands.

The Pacific ocean contains the some of the largest and most valuable tuna in the world.[17] Most small Pacific Island nations depend heavily on the ocean as their main source of economic development.[18] The question that should be asked, then, is how can these small island countries, who have no strong voice in the international community, compete with powerful countries such as the United States, Japan, or China, which have much better resources to conduct deep ocean fishing and have a stronger position in global trade? These powerful nations with resources for fishing deal with these small island countries of the Pacific as entities that are

---

15. Nathan Strout, "House committee moves South Pacific Tuna Treaty Act forward," Seafood Source, October 27, 2023, https://www.seafoodsource.com/news/supply-trade/house-committee-moves-south-pacific-tuna-treaty-act-forward forward.

16. Michael Di Girolamo, "Tuna Fisheries: A Cornerstone of US-Pacific Engagement," The Pacific Islands Matter for America Matters for Pacific Islands, February11, 2022, https://asiamattersforamerica.org/articles/tuna-fisheries-a-cornerstone-of-us-pacific-engagement.

17. Christopher Pale, "How Eight Pacific Island States are Saving the World's Tuna," FP, March 5, 2021, https://foreignpolicy.com/2021/03/05/tuna-fishing-overfishing-conservation-pacific-islands-skipjack-pna.

18. World Bank Group, "Pacific Islands: The Ocean Is Our Mother," August 29, 2012, https://www.worldbank.org/en/news/feature/2012/08/29/pacific-islands-the-ocean-is-our-mother; also UN Environment Programme, "Secretariat of the Pacific Environment Programme—The SPREP Convention," https://www.unep.org/explore-topics/oceans-seas/what-we-do/working-regional-seas/regional-seas-programmes/pacific#:~:text=Marine%20resources%20play%20a%20significant,landings%20come%20from%20Pacific%20waters.

unable to protect their ocean space and have no voice in international exchanges. For Pacific Islanders, the ocean is their home and should be treated with respect and care. It should not be treated as a commercial resource to be exploited for profit.

Canned fish from Asia and the United States currently provides most of the staple imports to the Pacific Islands, with the primary source coming from the same Pacific Ocean that surrounds these small island nations.[19] This could be compared with the situation the Indigenous tribes in the Pacific Northwest are facing, when the US government overfished the salmon from their rivers, poisoned them through mining and other illegal activities, and dammed rivers all the way up to the spawning grounds, causing the salmon to disappear.[20] The decline of salmon made it very expensive to buy fresh salmon. It forced some tribes to turn to canned salmon. Since the US Indigenous population is disproportionately affected by food insecurity, canned salmon is often part of the list of the products that they usually receive as part of free government commodities (rations).

CONCLUSION: RECOVERY AND REBUILDING IN THE PACIFIC

In response to the concerns related to dietary causes of NCDs, some Pacific Islands have challenged and changed the policies of free trade that make it easy for companies to penetrate the food markets and the food environments, especially those that promote distribution of processed foods that are high in salt, sugar, and fat.[21] However, in trying to create policies to combat that issue, policymakers face strong opposition from foreign food and beverage companies, which are trying to overturn these

---

19. Francisco Blaha, "The Canned Tuna Fishing Industry in the Pacific," blog, July 24, 2015,http://www.franciscoblaha.info/blog/2015/7/23/the-canned-tuna-fishing-industry. See also Transforming Tuna Fisheries in the Pacific, Nature Conservancy, https://www.nature.org/en-us/about-us/where-we-work/asia-pacific/the-pacific-islands/stories-in-the-pacific-islands/saving-tuna-¨populations-in-the-pacific/.

20. "Indigenous communities make their voices heard on climate and salmon," in *The Fig Tree* 41, 3, (March 2024), 9, http://www.thefigtree.org/march24/Mar24FT.pdf.

21. Thow et al., "Food trade among Pacific Island countries and territories.

policies. Islands of the Pacific have more recently worked to increase the promotion of sustainable agricultural practices and organic farming, instead of proclaiming that they are returning to Indigenous ways of farming. It is the Indigenous way of life to treat our ocean and our land with love and respect. It is time to bring back our Indigenous way of living and the knowledge that was by colonialists disqualified as unscientific and uncivilized.

In order to rediscover health in the Pacific, we need to work together. The more powerful countries should help the Pacific Islands correct the wrongs that they have done for many years. In addition, the United States, Japan, and China should stop their legal and illegal fishing in the Pacific Ocean and instead help the small Pacific Island nations access the ocean in a more sustainable way. There should be more regulations to decrease the availability and accessibility of unhealthy food and products. Also, governments should require clear warning statements and labeling to let consumers know the health risks associated with unhealthy foods.

Pacific Islands are small and have limited resources. In particular, they have little land for farming to provide food for the whole of their growing populations. This means that many of these islands may seek to rely on outside aid together with reviving the islands' own social and cultural ways of life, including Indigenous food cultures. Some scholars observe in Nauru that one Indigenous form of food sharing, which had been part of the islander's life and value, is taught to children from early age (McLennan and Ulijaszek 2015, 1499–1505).These young children were taught to give and share what they have. It is considered very bad manners not to share what you have. It became a part of the people's daily life. However, this life value was replaced after their contacted with the colonizers.

Pacific Islanders need incentives to revive our Indigenous food system which will not only improve our diets but also strengthen our community connections. Strengthening the community connection allows opportunity for different generations to share knowledges and resources. As part of the traditions that I grew up with in Tonga, every Sunday every house would prepare good dishes for their neighbors. In doing so, we had an opportunity to share with our neighbors the good food we ate that Sunday.

As a kid, I always looked forward to eating the good dishes from our neighbors. Our continued survival is based on a belief in inter-dependence, that we are dependent on each other. Our agricultural life is threatened by climate change and by commercialization and outside interests in profit over people's lives. Returning to indigenous ways of farming and fishing and our own local food systems will help Pacific Islanders overcome these dietary diseases and enable us to return to a healthier balance of living and eating.

17

Food Crises
Rereading Numbers 11 in and with Moana Worldviews

Jione Havea

FOOD NOURISHES BODIES as well as relationships. In the (proverbial) old days, in ancient Pasifika (for Pacific, Oceania),[1] food was the staple (foodstuff, fastener) that bound individuals, families, and communities to each other, and to their island worlds. Put differently, food was the yoke (pun intended) between Pasifika natives, other kinds of island dwellers (occupiers, settlers), and their island worlds. Pasifika natives live in relation with four worlds: (is)land, sea, sky, and underworld. And in the language of modern folx, food is currency (in contrast to commodity).

This *talanoa* is food for thought on the significance of food in Pasifika—drawing on the *wun-tok* culture of so-called Melanesian[2] Islanders—and

1. Pasifika (alt. Pasefika, Pasifiki, etc.) is one of the Indigenous renderings of the label "Pacific" that Europeans gave to our waters and islands. I use the term as a reminder of our colonial history, a history that has not ended.

2. I say "so-called" because "Melanesia" is the name that European navigators and scholars gave to the group of islands in the mid-west of Pasifika, because their native peoples were black/mela. This group includes Papua New Guinea, West Papua (occupied by Indonesia),

how that shapes a Moana reading of the food crises narrated in Numbers 11. *Talanoa* is the confluence (or intersecting) of three fluxes: a gift (of intersecting stories); an act (of telling and talking); and an event (of listening and then conversing and exchanging, with elements of interrogation and some pushing back). Food is corporal and social currency, but can it also be hermeneutical currency? This is the meta-critical question that lurks behind this talanoa.

MOANA

I draw upon the *won-tok* culture to develop a reading of Numbers 11 that is undertaken in and with native island worlds ((is)land, sea, sky, underworld); that is, a reading in and with Moana worldviews. The Moana reading offered here represents the current state of biblical criticisms in Pasifika (which i[3] sketch below). This is one but not my only attempt to craft Moana reading, and other Pasifika natives will join our craft/canoe at their pace and space.

Won-tok

Won-tok is the name that so-called Melanesian Islanders give to people who speak a form of creole/pidgin language, because those people share "one talk."[4] While each community has a native tongue that they share with other communities in their kinship clan, the pidgin *won-tok* language allows them to communicate outside of their first (clan, kinship) language. It is therefore expected of won-tok natives to be bilingual. The pidgin/creole

---

Solomon Islands, Vanuatu, Kanaky (New Caledonia, occupied by France), and Fiji—each island group has diverse and rich customs that cannot be reduced to some common cultural denominator. Referring to this group as Melanesian, as if they are "one people," is unjust.

3. I use the lowercase "i" (except at the beginning of a sentence) because i also use the lowercase with you, she, we, he, they, it, and other. This is a sign of my affirmation that i (as individual) do not exist without relating to others and to the surroundings, a sign of my resistance against the privileging of the so-called independent modern self, and a sign of my rebellion against the colonial English language.

4. At this juncture, i confess to the obvious: i am a native of the Tonga Islands, which is outside and southeast of the so-called Melanesian Islands. Won-tok is not a term in the Tongan vocabulary, but we understand and embody the won-tok culture.

language is their second language. They may also understand and speak other native languages due to the multiple belongings of their parents, their marriage to other clans and islands, the location of their place of schooling or employment, and several other factors.

The *won-tok* people include natives from the Solomon Islands, West Papua, Papua New Guinea, and Vanuatu. The *won-tok* language is necessary for them because there are many living languages in each group. There are more than sixty native languages still spoken in the Solomon Islands, more than 140 native languages spoken in Vanuatu, and more than 830 native languages spoken across West Papua and Papua New Guinea. *Won-tok* natives can also communicate across the three main forms of pidgin/creole: Pijin in Solomon Islands, Tok-Pisin in Papua New Guinea and West Papua, and Bislama in Vanuatu. The *won-tok* people are clever natives.

Across cultural and island borders, the *won-tok* natives may not be related by heritage or kinship, but sharing the same *tok* ("talk" in creole) makes them relatives—*won-tok*—obliging them to care for one another as members of a "*won-tok* household." In the *won-tok* culture, a household is not limited to a family, village, clan, or tribe. Rather, a household extends to other people who can communicate and understand one another. *Won-tok* is Pentecost-like (see Acts 2).

Solomon Island elder and theologian Leslie Boseto interweaves the *won-tok* custom with the theological understanding of the English term "household" (from two Greek words: *oikos*/house + *nomos*/custom) in his conception of *won-tok* economy (Boseto 1995, 179–184).[5] A household functions according to a won-tok form of "economy" (also: oikos/eco + nomos), and food is the critical component at the center of won-tok interactions. Tribal territories and rights are defined, regulated, and challenged for food security. Discords and wars, marriages and treaties, covenants and alliances, are dis/established with and for the sake of securing food.

Food is the currency in *won-tok* economy, and economy is the *staple* (feed, adhesive) in the *won-tok* household/culture. Food is valuable not because it is a product to be traded and turned into profit, but because it

5. There was no Pasifika voice in the first edition of *Voices from the Margin*. Boseto's essay was added to the second edition but removed from the third and later editions.

is the currency that makes the *won-tok* economy tick. Put another way, food feeds, inspires, and empowers *oikos* + *nomos* (Havea 2024, np).

Won-tok customs anticipate the sharing of space, resources, and collaboration for the sake of food.[6] In this context, the *won-tok* economy does not function according to capitalist currencies and valuations but in line with responsibilities and services, and Boseto brings this custom into the realm of theology:

> Gospel and economy belong together. Both good news (gospel) and economy are related to creation. Our ancestors located their gods in creation. Their gods resided in the rivers, the mountains, valley, reefs, trees, and so forth. They were not far away and above us in heaven (Boseto 1995, 180).

The *won-tok* economy functions at the intersection of relationships (*vā*, *wā*: partnership between human- and other-kinds) and responsibilities (*tautua*: service, labor). Boseto is thus critical of people who benefit from the modern, capitalist economy: "Yet many people today want to rape our mother-earth for their own use, for their own benefits, without recognizing our real cousins, brothers and sisters within the one world-household" (Boseto 1995, 182).

Moana Biblical Criticisms

Moana biblical criticisms represent the confluence of three hermeneutical movements that have been rippling across and from Pasifika: Pacific hermeneutics, island(er) criticisms, and native criticisms (see also Havea, forthcoming). I joined the first of these movements over thirty years ago, and i hope that future generations of Pasifika biblical critics will give them new energies and *niu* (one of the terms for "coconut," referring to something local) directions.

To use another oceanic metaphor, Moana biblical criticism is like a lagoon in which, on this occasion, three biblical hermeneutical crafts/canoes harbor. Pacific hermeneutics was the first canoe, launched before my time, and it called attention to the ways and wisdoms of our local Pasifika region,

6. When sharing does not take place, conflicts erupt.

with the intention that they would help us read biblical texts in our island-worlds.[7] The second is island(er) criticisms set out during my time in the context of the Society of Biblical Literature and reached into the Caribbean waters and other island settings, such as imperial islands in Europe and Asia. We have been intentional in collaboratively publishing and in forming *won-tok* relations, pushing our canoe into the wharfs of dominant white and whitish scholarship.[8] The third is native criticisms set out more recently, with the courage to flip at (give the middle finger) as well as flip (turn over) colonial scriptures and colonialist mindsets.[9] These three Pasifika hermeneutical canoes meet up at Moana biblical criticisms.

I don't use the labels "contextual" or "Indigenous" interpretations because, in and from Pasifika worldviews, those are empty boxes assigned by dominant white and whitish scholars for those of us who do things differently. The "contextual" and "Indigenous" labels are part of the colonial project.[10] Put sharply, they are labels for boxes that dominant white and whitish scholars built to deny the differences between *minoritized scholars* in white societies as well as between *real scholars* from Africa, Asia, America, Caribbean, and Pasifika. I don't jump into those white and whitish boxes; rather, i prefer to get into canoes that we built for ourselves—namely, Pacific hermeneutics, island(er) criticisms, native criticisms, and now Moana criticisms. These are native canoes for which we use our native stuff, and we built them in our ways to deliver our answers to our questions (instead of answering someone else's questions, for their (neo)colonial causes).

Moana Worldviews

Moana biblical criticisms are also like a lagoon into which the world and worldviews of native Pasifika Island(er)s flow. Like for all other people,

7. See, e.g., Havea 2003; Vaka'uta 2011; Nofoaiga 2017; Mailo 2016; Havea and Lau 2020; Havea 2021d; Kolia forthcoming.

8. See, e.g., Havea, Neville, and Wainwright 2014; Havea, Aymer, and Davidson 2015; Havea 2018.

9. See, e.g., Havea 2021a, 82–89; Havea 2021a, 349–57.

10. Similar to the way that the tags "Polynesia," "Micronesia," and "Melanesia" are used to categorize and homogenize the diverse groups of native Pasifika island(er)s.

our worldviews are shaped by our worlds, and thus, our worldviews are different in details among the various island groups, because no two islands are the same. However, the diverse Pasifika Island groups share the recognition of at least three of the following four living bodies in our island worlds: (is)land/*fenua*, sea/*wasa*, sky/*langi*, and underworld/*pulotu*. Three of these bodies—*fenua*, *wasa*, *langi*—are visible, but the unseen *pulotu* is hauntingly ever-present in the three visible bodies. We have different names for these bodies, but they are recognized across Pasifika cultures. Moreover, natives think and expect these bodies to be connected—in other words, to be *won-tok*.

I use the label Moana for the meeting of the four bodies. At this juncture, i flip at Disney: Disney messed things up when their 2016 animation titled *Moana*, the name for the brave and playful young woman character, is also presented as the name for the sea. In the Pasifika worlds, Moana is one of the names for the deep, dark blue sea—far from the (is)land. We have other names for the shallow part of the sea (for example, in Tongan: *namo*, *fanga*, *liku*), and other names for the whole ocean—i use the Fijian term *wasa* (*vasa* in Samoan, *vaha* in Tongan) in this talanoa. For this talanoa, i use *wasa* for the whole ocean and Moana for the meeting of the four bodies of the Pasifika worldviews.

When i (re)tell native sacred stories, i draw attention to the meeting of the four bodies of the Moana worldviews. For instance, in one of the Tongan sacred creation stories, there were only Moana (deep, blue sea) and pulotu at the beginning, before creation began. Then fire came up from pulotu to form an island; followed by a bird coming from the sky with a seed that dropped onto the island and grew into a creeper, from which came a maggot that was severed (by the same bird) into three pieces. The three pieces of the maggot turned into three human beings—Kohai was female, Koau was male, and Momo was of the third gender—and Maui brought partners for them from Pulotu, and they populated the island with native Tongans. According to this ancient talanoa, the creation of the Tonga group was through the collaboration between pulotu (underworld), sea, sky, and fenua ((is)land). These four island bodies are co-creators—with the help of a bird and the sacrifice of a maggot.

The collaboration between these co-creators is an example of *won-tok* culture. The four bodies have different features and textures (read: *tok*) specific for their own space, but they become won/one in creation.

MOANA READING

In light of the sacred creation talanoa above, to read in and with Moana worldviews involves reading (1) for the presence and (2) for the *won-tok* engagement of the four bodies in the island worlds: (is)land, sea, sky, underworld. The first task can be easily carried out with texts like Genesis 1:1–2, because the four bodies are plainly named or inferred:

> When God began to create the heavens [sky] and the earth [(is)land], 2 the earth was complete chaos, and darkness covered the face of the deep [underworld], while a wind from God swept over the face of the waters [sea]. (NRSVue; annotations added)

However, the four bodies are not named as present in most biblical texts, and there is a simple explanation for this: biblical texts are from a different world. Nonetheless, one could undertake a Moana reading of texts where the four bodies are not named. Take for instance the Shema' (Deuteronomy 6:4–7), over which identifying the four Moana bodies will involve some *won-tok*-ing:

> 4 "Hear, O Israel: The LORD is our God, the LORD alone. 5 You shall love the LORD your God with all your heart and with all your soul and with all your might. 6 Keep these words that I am commanding you today in your heart. 7 Recite them to your children and talk about them when you are at home [(is)land] and when you are away [at sea], when you lie down [and look up to the sky] and when you rise [and look down to the underworld]. 8 Bind them as a sign on your hand, fix them as an emblem on your forehead, 9 and write them on the doorposts of your house and on your gates. (NRSVue; annotations added).

The LORD did not locate the Shema' at the four bodies of the island worlds, but those bodies are also implied in the explanations that follow:

underworld—the home of the ancestors—is implied in the identifying of Abraham, Isaac, and Jacob as ancestors in verse 10; *sky* is implied in the reference to Massah in verse 16, because the LORD was positioned above/skyward on the rock at Horeb (Exodus 17:6); *(is)land* is named in verse 18; and *sea* is implied in the reference to the people that the Shema' addresses as being brought out of Egypt—across the Sea of Reeds—in verse 21.

Identifying the four bodies of the island worlds in the Shema' involve a *won-tok* exercise. To read the Shema' with Moana worldviews (the second task, which i reserve for another occasion) will involve a hermeneutical leap. This is not a bizarre admission, because all readers take hermeneutical leaps into the worlds of meanings behind, within, in front of, besides, and under biblical texts. Biblical criticism is an art of *won-tok*-ing and taking hermeneutical leaps, with the help of traditional and nontraditional methods and worldviews.

Food

One of the points at which the four bodies of Pasifika worldviews meet is food—we consume creatures from the sea, from the land, from the sky, and from the underworld. And at the end of our journey, our bodies will be consumed by creatures and forces who will return our remains to the (is)land, sea, sky, and underworld.

While alive, the foodstuff that we raise, whether we are vegetarian, carnivore, or some variation of both, depends on the waters that come up from the (is)land, on the energies that the moon and stars send, on the minerals that come from the sea and the underworld, on the wind that carries air and sustenance across the sky, sea, and (is)lands, and on the mercy and hospitality of the (is)lands. No human person can raise and yield food without the presence and assistance of the four bodies of the Pasifika worldviews. The *won-tok* spirit plays out in the collaboration of the four bodies on the yielding of food.

Assuming, of course, that the four bodies are healthy, willing, and cooperating. In this regard, lack of food is evidence that something has gone awry in the *won-tok* relationship between the four bodies. This is the condition that we find in stories of famine (for example, Genesis 12, 26, 41; Ruth 1; 2 Samuel 21) as well as in Numbers 11—something has gone awry.

NUMBERS 11

Numbers 11 opens with the people complaining,[11] and the LORD getting so mad that they[12] burned the people with fire (11:1–3). The text locates the fire with the LORD (v. 1), whose anger and wrath make their face or presence fiery. In the biblical worldview, this kind of fire is associated with the (hot) breath of the LORD.

In ancient talanoa, on the other hand, Pasifika worldviews locate fire in the underworld (*pulotu*), and it has creative energy. And in current times, what has been called the Pacific Ring of Fire is evidence that a sea of fire flow under our feet. I call attention to the difference in worldviews as a signal that a Moana reading may be different from, and may even subvert, the biblical LORD's agenda and cause.

The cause of the people's complaint is not stated, but it resulted in "hardships" (NIV) or "misfortunes" (NRSVue), and there is a hint that the people complained publicly and may have thus caused the LORD to lose face. The people banged, and the Lord boomed and burned. From the outset, the LORD's extreme response suggests that the people were dealing with a tyrant, or a monster, who did not like people who talk and push back.

Food

The LORD's response was to burn the people, and the place was given a name—Tabera/burning—as a reminder of what happened. But burning the people publicly did not resolve anything. The people cried to Moses. Moses interceded, and the fire abated. After some time, the people came back with another complaint, this time relating to food:

---

11. Complaining is a key feature in the wilderness narrative, which spreads from the book of Exodus to the book of Deuteronomy and has been used by tradition-critics to justify the rejection of the generation that was liberated from Egypt as a rebellious lot. The event at Massah (previously named Rephidim) noted in the Shema' was in response to the people complaining. On that occasion, the people complained because there was no water to drink (Exodus 17:1–7).

12. I follow the Qur'anic tradition of using the third person plural for the deity. This scriptural tradition affirms the call for inclusive language from feminist and *takatāpui*/LGBTQ+ folx.

> If only we had meat to eat! 5 We remember the fish we used to eat in Egypt *for nothing*, the cucumbers, the melons, the leeks, the onions, and the garlic, 6 but now our strength is dried up, and there is nothing at all but this manna to look at. (NRSVue, my italics)

This time around, the people's complaint was due to the lack of meat and vegetables. This complaining lot was accustomed to eating well in Egypt, at no cost or limit to them, which suggests that they were not regular slaves like the estimated twelve-plus million black African slaves that were abducted by white, majority Christian slave traders in the Atlantic slave trade. I do not hear in the complaint of this lot the kind of desperation that i see in the faces of poor and displaced people, from the streets of first-world nations to modern open-air prisons (like Gaza) and fields of war (from Haiti to Ukraine and across to Myanmar, Ethiopia, Sudan, and other poorer nations).

As a co-parent, i hear this kind of complaint almost every day. And i often get angry, but not so angry that i would consider burning our privileged middle-class daughter. So i understand the people's complaint, even if they belonged to the privileged upper class, but i am disappointed with the LORD's extreme, ungodly response—to burn the people, the children, who were dependent on them. The God who was expected to sustain and liberate did not do as expected.[13]

Moses interceded on behalf of the people and pushed the Lord to be a responsible parent. The LORD's response went to the other extreme:

> Therefore the LORD will give you meat, and you shall eat. 19 You shall eat not only one day, or two days, or five days, or ten days, or twenty days, 20 but for a whole month, *until it comes out of your nostrils and becomes loathsome to you*—because you have rejected the Lord who is among you and have wailed before him, saying, "Why did we ever leave Egypt?" (NRSVue, my italics)

The people were longing for fish and vegetables (as in Egypt), and the LORD promised to give them lots and lots of meat. Either the LORD did

---

13. See also De La Torre, forthcoming.

not hear the people properly, or the LORD has a cruel sense of humor. The LORD's solution, which reads like Moses' plot, is not a satisfying solution. It made things worse for the craving people. They are to eat meat (but no vegetables were provided) until they puke. The LORD was still very angry. Nasty. Unparentlike. Horrible.

Why this cruelty? The people seem to have touched a raw nerve: according to the LORD, as Moses explained, the people questioned why they ever left Egypt (v. 20). At that point in the narrative, Moses and the Lord would have been proud that they liberated the people from Egypt. But then, the people gave the impression that they may have been *made to leave* Egypt (without consultation; without their consent): "Why did we ever leave Egypt?" This was the impression that Moses gave as justification for the LORD's cruel response to their complaint.

The alternative food came in the form of quails, which came up from the sea. The LORD sent a wind across the sky, to bring birds from the sea.

> 31 Then a wind went out from the LORD, and it brought quails from the sea and let them fall beside the camp, about a day's journey on this side and a day's journey on the other side, all around the camp, about two cubits deep on the ground.

A MOANA READING

The solution for the complaint of the people who were on the (is)land, in the wilderness, came up from the sea, through the sky. In this inter-action, three of the four bodies of the Pasifika worldviews are involved.

The fourth body is inferred: The wind was sent by the LORD, the same angry character who earlier burned the people with fire, which, in the biblical worldview, comes from the presence or face of the LORD. In Moana worldviews, on the other hand, as explained above, fire is energy that comes from *pulotu*, from the underworld—the fourth body of the Pasifika worldviews.

At this juncture of crafting a Moana reading, the four bodies—(is)land, sea, sky, and underworld—are present in Numbers 11, and the LORD is the angry character that crosses and messes things up—first, by throwing fire at the children of Israel; then the LORD killed more birds than needed—unnecessary waste; and the story ended with a plague that sent more people to the home of the ancestors. The LORD is the destructive and wasteful character in this story of food crisis.[14]

SO WHAT?

In the face of food crises, people tend to look for someone or some reason to blame: We didn't prepare the ground appropriately, our seedlings were not healthy, we didn't plant at the right time, or there were extended droughts and extreme weathers due to climate change. And in the global context, for instance, Putin's invasion of Ukraine is causing food shortages in Africa and raising the cost of living across the world. There are many other reasons, but rarely do people lay the blame at the feet of divine beings.

Numbers 11, on the other hand, makes clear that the reckless and wasteful deity—the LORD—is causing the food crises. My aim here is not to expose the deity of the Hebrew Bible as a reckless and wasteful deity; the texts of the Hebrew Bible do that on their own. Nor is my aim to portray the deity of the Hebrew Bible as being more reckless and wasteful than the deity of the Christian Bible: Jesus—the son of God in the Christian Bible—was also cruel with such teachings as "If your hand causes you to stumble, cut it off; it is better for you to enter life maimed than to have two hands and to go to Gehenna, to the unquenchable fire" (Mark 9:43).

Rather, my aim in this talanoa is to call attention to how the sovereign deity of the Bible—the LORD—disrespected and mistreated the four bodies of the Moana worldviews. Such was the case in Numbers 11, and the result was food crisis. To that i add that the next time we want to blame someone or something for food crises, we should begin by asking if anyone or anything—divine, human, living, or artificial—has been disrespectful against and mistreated (is)land, sea, sky, and underworld. I suggest this not because i wish to fix the blame for food crises on anything, but because i pray that we are more respectful of (the four bodies of) the Moana worldviews.

---

14. Up to this point, my aim has been to identify the four Moana bodies in Numbers 11. I will continue crafting the Moana reading in my forthcoming commentary on Numbers for the Wisdom Commentary Series of Liturgical Press.

CONTRIBUTORS

Yvette R. Blair-Lavallais is a faith leader, food justice scholar, and ecowomanist situated in Dallas. She earned her Doctor of Ministry in "Land, Food, and Faith Formation" at Memphis Theological Seminary, where she also serves as an adjunct faculty member teaching Theology of the Land. As a community pastor, Yvette amplifies her voice at the intersection of faith and food injustice. She presents at conferences domestically and globally and is the 2024–25 Equity Research Fellow with Feeding America.

Anugrah Brij is currently in his third year of theological studies at Bishop's College, Kolkata. He holds an MA in English Literature from St. Stephen's College, Delhi. Preparing for ordained ministry in the Church of North India, he is deeply interested in Dalit Theology and Indian Church History.

Kalzang Dorjee Bhutia is originally from western Sikkim, India, and completed his PhD in Buddhist studies at Delhi University. His research has been supported by an ACLS/Robert H. N. Ho Research Fellowship in Buddhist studies, the American Council for Learned Societies, and the Wenner Gren Foundation. He is currently completing a monograph on the environmental history of Buddhism in Sikkim.

Miguel A. De La Torre, is an international scholar, documentarian, novelist, academic author, and scholar activist. Since obtaining his doctoral in 1999, he has authored more than a hundred articles and published forty-seven books (six of which won national awards). He currently serves as professor of Social Ethics and Latine Studies at the Iliff School of Theology in Denver. A Fulbright scholar, he has served as the 2012 president of the Society of Christian Ethics. He is the recipient of the 2020 AAR Excellence in Teaching Award and the 2021 Martin E. Marty Public Understanding of Religion Award. Recently, he wrote the screenplay to a documentary on immigration that has won more than seven awards. Additionally, he has written an autofiction magical realism novel.

'Ikani Fakasi'i'eiki is an ordained elder of the Free Wesleyan Church of Tonga, a member of Liberty Park UMC. He is a community health worker, working with homeless families through Catholic Charities of Eastern Washington. He studied at Sia'atoutai Theological College in Tonga (BD), Pacific Theological College in Suva, Fiji (MTh), and Pacific School of Religion/Graduate Theological Union (MABL). He received his PhD from the Graduate Theological Union in Berkeley, California. He taught at Sia'atoutai Theological College and lectured at Eastern Washington University in Cheney and Gonzaga University in Spokane, Washington. His research interests include the Hebrew Bible, postcolonial/colonial discourse analysis, Oceanic/Pacific Islander perspectives, and climate change and the Pacific.

Jione Havea is co-parent for Diya Lākai, native pastor (Methodist Church in Tonga), migrant to the cluster of islands now known as Australia, and senior research fellow with Trinity Methodist Theological College (Aotearoa New Zealand) and with Centre for Religion, Ethics, and Society (Charles Sturt University, Australia). Jione is energized by opportunities to collaborate and excuses for theological (broadly conceived) revol-u-ting.

Steven James is working towards his PhD in Religion and Politics at the University of Denver and Iliff School of Theology's Joint Doctoral Program in the Study of Religion. Steven researches religious social movements, intersectional politics, decolonial thought, liberative theologies and ethics, Latine/x cultures and histories, and LGBTQ+ issues.

Lynnette Xiangling Li, is a doctoral student at the University of Denver ILIFF School of Theology's joint PhD program. Their academic interests include postcolonial studies, environmental ethics, Ecodharma, and liberative theologies. They have published work around environmental vulnerability and hazardous mitigation. They are a doctoral fellow with the Louisville Institute and an academic fellow with the Council for World Mission.

Terence Mupangwa is an academic scholar in religion and gender. Since obtaining her doctoral in 2022, she has authored five book chapters and two journal articles. She is currently a postdoctoral research fellow at the University of Cape Town in South Africa. Before coming to the University of Cape Town she held lectureship posts at two universities in Zimbabwe, Catholic University and Women's University in Africa, respectively.

Jessica Ordaz is an assistant professor of Ethnic Studies at the University of Colorado Boulder. Her first book, *The Shadow of El Centro: A History of Migrant Incarceration and Solidarity*, was released in March 2021. Her second project will explore the multifaceted history of veganism and plant-based foods throughout the Americas, focusing on colonization, food politics, and social justice. This research will illuminate the wider and transnational history of Latinx veganism and how communities of color have engaged with questions of animal, human, and plant relations for centuries.

Bianca Mendes Rati was born and raised Brazilian and is one of the founders of the *Projeto Redomas*, a digital activism organization that works against misogyny, racism, and LGBTQ+phobia within Christian spaces, especially evangelical spaces, through content production such as podcasts, texts, Bible studies, and booklets. She has a degree in graphic design and a master's degree in design from the Federal University of Paraná, with a focus on gender, philosophy, and visuality. Bianca got involved with environment and animal activism after realizing how all oppressions are connected and that there's no true liberation if we are not all liberated.

Kigéw Puri (André da Silva Muniz) is seed of the Puri people. She graduated in Theology with a specialization in Anthropology and is a master's student in Human and Social Sciences. Her research revolves around the intersectionality between gender and sexuality diversity among Indigenous peoples and, more specifically, her own ethnicity, the Puri.

Taimaya Ragui is a tribal-Indigenous researcher from Ukhrul, Northeast India. He has a PhD in theology from the South Asia Institute of Advanced Christian Studies. After completing his doctoral study, he has been conducting research on decolonial studies, such as decolonial theology, spirituality, and mission. Currently, he serves as a research tutor at the Shepherd's Academy of Oxford Centre for Religion and Public Life.

Dennis Saavedra Carquin-Hamichand is a PhD student at the Iliff School of Theology and the University of Denver in the Religious Studies Joint Doctoral Program. His research is centered on suicide prevention and intervention in Guyana, employing decolonial, ethical, and social justice frameworks. He is the Graduate Student Association (GSA) president for the JDP's 2023–24 academic year. He is a two-time recipient of the Elizabeth Iliff Warren Scholarship (2021 and 2022) and a 2023 recipient of the Luce-AAR Advancing Public Scholarship.

Hesron H. Sihombing is a doctoral student at the University of Denver Iliff School of Theology. An Indonesian native of the Batak ethnic group, he has authored articles published in the *International Journal of Public Theology*, *CrossCurrents*, *Siwó*, and other venues. His main interests lie at the intersection of liberative ethics, public theology, postcolonial studies, and economic and ecological issues. His current research examines the ethical and postcolonial perspectives of the digital economy.

Aline Silva has served for more than a decade as a local parish pastor of rural and farming populations in Kansas, Missouri, and Colorado. Most recently she served as the executive director of a Farmed Animal Welfare organization. Aline shares herself as a queer, Black, and Indigenous immigrant of *Brasil* to the United States. Aline chooses not to eat nonhuman animals, her fellow-worshippers of God. Aline is an organizer, pastor, preacher, and life coach. She writes today from the unceded lands of the Tequesta, Taíno, and Seminole peoples, namely South Florida, USA.

Sonakshi Srivastava is a senoir writing tutor at Ashoka University, Sonepat, India. She previously graduated from the University of Delhi, where she read English Literature. Her MPhil dissertation was on the biopolitics of ability and debility in contemporary fiction. She is a resident researcher for ForeignObjekt and one of the recipients of South Asia Speaks mentorship programme, working on translating the Hindi novel *Titli* into English. She was also shortlisted for the 2020 Serendipity FoodLab Residency and was a Tempus Public Foundation Fellow in 2021. Her works have previously appeared in or are appearing in the Bilingual Window, ASAP Connect, Hakara, potluck zine, orangepeel mag, and Rhodora, among others. She is widely passionate about discard studies, food literatures, astromancy, posthumanism, zines, and animal studies.

tink tinker is a citizen of the Osage Nation (*wazhazhe udsethe*) and emeritus professor of American Indian studies at iliff school of theology. As an academic, tinker is committed to a scholarly endeavor that takes seriously both the liberation of Indian Peoples from their historic oppression as colonized communities and the liberation of eurochristian americans, the historic colonizers and oppressors of Indian Peoples. A scholar/activist, tinker has worked closely with both Four Winds American Indian Council in denver and the American Indian Movement of colorado. He has written several books and nearly a hundred journal articles and chapters.

Bernardo R. Vargas is a philosopher whose primary area of research centers on questions of oppression and liberation, particularly regarding racial identity, racism, and environmental justice as they relate to Mexican Americans and Latinxs in the United States. He is a Crossing Latinidades Mellon Humanities Fellow in the Climate and Environmental Justice Crossing Latinidades Humanities Research Working Group, which aims to reveal how Latina/o/x communities confront environmental injustices and adapt to extreme climate events. He is also a PhD candidate of Philosophy and a teaching fellow for the Philosophy and Religion department at the University of North Texas.

BIBLIOGRAPHY

Abbott, Elizabeth. 2009. *Sugar: A Bittersweet History*. London: Duckworth.

Ackerman, Rudi Michiel. 2017. *Financialisation in South African Agriculture: Two Firm-Level Case Studies*. Johannesburg: University of the Witwatersrand.

Adams, Francis. 2020. *The Right to Food: The Global Campaign to End Hunger and Malnutrition*. Cham: Palgrave Macmillan.

Alatas, Seyd Hussein. 1977. *The Myth of the Lazy Native: A Study of the Image of the Malays, Filipinos and Javanese from the 16th to 20th Century and Its Function in the Ideology of Colonial Capitalism*. London: Frank Cass.

Albala, Ken. 2014. *From Famine to Fast Food: Nutrition, Diet, and Concepts of Health Around the World*. London: Bloomsbury.

Ali, Asim, and Patrick Schena. 2017. "Look Before You Leap: Weighing the Consequences of a Sovereign Wealth Fund Aimed at Harnessing Oil Resources in Guyana." *Harvard International Review* 38(4): 23–24.

Ali, Grace Aneiza. 2020. *Liminal Spaces: Migration and Women of the Guyanese Diaspora*. Cambridge, UK: Open Book.

Ambedkar, Bhim Rao. 1946. "Hindu Social Order." In *Writings and Speeches* 3: 106–113.

_______. 2014. "*India and the Prerequisites of Communism*." In *Dr. Babasaheb Ambedkar: Writings and Speeches*, 3. Edited by Vasant Moon. Delhi: Dr. Ambedkar Foundation.

Andersen, Martin Edwin. 2010. *Peoples of the Earth: Ethnonationalism, Democracy, and the Indigenous Challenge in 'Latin' America*. Blue Ridge Summit: Rowman & Littlefield.

Asnewastri. 2018. "Migrasi Etnik Batak Toba Ke Nagori Mariah Bandar Kecamatan Pematang Bandar, 1946–2011." *Sejarah Dan Budaya: Jurnal Sejarah, Budaya, Dan Pengajarannya* 12, no.1 (June): 8–18.

Bahadur, Gaiutra. 2013. *Coolie Woman: The Odyssey of Indenture*. Gurgaon, IND: Hachette India.

Balston, C. 2020. *The Amazon's mouth-watering 'fifth flavour.'* https://www.bbc.com/travel/article/20201122-the-amazons-mouth-watering-fifth-flavour.

Baragwanath, Kathryn, and Ella Bayi. 2020. "Collective Property Rights Reduce Deforestation in the Brazilian Amazon." *Proceedings of the National Academy of Sciences* 117, no. 34 (August 25): 22495–20502.

Baron, Robert, and Ana C. Cara. 2011. *Creolization as Cultural Creativity* 1st Ed. Jackson: University Press of Mississippi.

Barbora, Sanjay, Bengt G. Karlsson, Dolly Kikon, Dixita Deka, Meenal Tula, and Joel Rodrigues. 2023. "Introduction." In *Seeds and Food Sovereignty*. Edited by Dixita Deka, Joel Rodrigues, Dolly Kikon, Bengt G. Karlsson, Sanjay Barbora, and Meenal Tula. Guwahati, IND: North Eastern Social Research Centre.

Bhabha, H. K. 2004. *The Location of Culture*. New York: Routledge.

Bhattacharjee, Nilanjana. 2019. "Lived Realities of Women Sanitation Workers in India: Insights from a Participatory Research Conducted in Three Cities of India." In *Participatory Research in Asia, New Delhi, India*. New Delhi: Participatory Research in Asia.

Bhutia, Kalzang Dorjee. 2021a. "Purifying Multispecies Relations in the Valley of Abundance: The *Riwo Sangchö* Ritual as Environmental History and Ethics in Sikkim," MAVCOR 5, no. 2 (2021a): 10.22332/mav.ess.2021.1.

______. 2021b. "Living with the Mountain: Mountain Propitiation Rituals as Pedagogy for Human-Environment Relations in Sikkim." *Journal of Buddhist Ethics* 28 (2021b): 261–94.

______. 2022. "Ignoring the Protectors: Slipping Soil and Relations in Village Resettlement Projects in the West Sikkim Himalayas." In

Shifting Climates, Shifting People. Edited by Miguel A. De La Torre. Cleveland: Pilgrim Press, 2022.

Bhuyan, Deep Jyoti et al. 2014. "Biochemical and Nutritional Analysis of Rice Beer of North East India." *Indian Journal of Traditional Knowledge* 13:1 (2014): 142–148.

Bilby, Kenneth. 1989. Review of "Linguistic Anthropology: Dimensions of a Creole Continuum: History, Texts, and Linguistic Analysis of Guyanese Creole" by John R. Rickford. *American Anthropologist*, 91, no. 1 (March 1989): 264–265. https://doi.org/10.1525/aa.1989.91.1.02a00920.

Boff, Leonardo, and Clodovis Boff. 1988. *Salvation and Liberation: In Search of a Balance between Faith and Politics*. Maryknoll, N.Y: Orbis Books.

Bollard, A. E. 1981. "The Financial Adventures of J. C. Godeffroy and Son in the Pacific." *The Journal of Pacific History* 16, no. 1 (January): 3–19.

Borah, Tasvina R., R. Helim, Robin Gogoi, and Ashok Kumar. 2012. "Versatile Uses of Maize in Sikkim." *Asian Agri-History* 16, no. 2: 211–15.

Boseto, Leslie. 1995. "The Gospel of Economy from a Solomon Islands Perspective." In *Voices from the Margin: Interpreting the Bible in the Third World*, 2nd ed. Edited by R. S. Sugirtharajah. Maryknoll: Orbis Books.

Boxer, Charles R. 2007. *A Igreja militante e a expansão ibérica 1440–1770*. Translated by Vera Maria Pereira. São Paulo: Companhia das Letras.

Bradley, Katharine, and Hank Herrera. 2016. "Decolonizing Food Justice: Naming, Resisting, and Researching Colonizing Forces in the Movement." *Antipode* 48: 97–114.

Bristol, Laurette. 2023. "Foreword." In *The Movement of Venezuelans to the Americas and the Caribbean in the 21st Century*. Edited by Wendell C. Wallace. Palgrave Macmillan.

Brueck, Julia Feliz. 2017. *Veganism in an Oppressive World: A Vegans of Color Community Project*. Coppell, Sanctuary Publishers, 2017.

Bureau of Statistics. 2016. *Final 2012 Census Compendium 2—Population Composition*. https://statisticsguyana.gov.gy/census/.

Burkhart, Brian. 2019. *Indigenizing Philosophy through the Land: A Trickster Methodology for Decolonizing Environmental Ethics and Indigenous Futures*. East Lansing: Michigan State University Press.

Byman, Daniel, and Jennifer Lind. 2010. "Pyongyang's Survival Strategy: Tools of Authoritarian Control in North." *International Security* 35, no. 1: 44–74.

Calvin, Linda, Philip Martin, and Skyler Simnitt. 2022. *Adjusting to Higher Labor Costs in Selected U.S. Fresh Fruit and Vegetable Industries*. Washington D.C.: U.S. Department of Agriculture.

Canettieri, Thiago. 2022. "O devir-periferia do mundo: crise do capital e a condição periférica." GEOgraphia 24, no. 52 (March 30): 1–18.

Carter-Pokras, Olivia, Ruth E. Zambrana, Carolyn F. Poppell, Laura A. Logie, and Rafael Guerrero-Preston. 2007. "The Environmental Health of Latino Children." Journal of Pediatric Health Care: *Official Publication of National Association of Pediatric Nurse Associates & Practitioners* 21, no. 5: 307–14.

Césaire, Aimé. 2000. *Discourse on Colonialism*. New York: Monthly Review Press.

Chao, Sophie. 2022. "Gastrocolonialism: The Intersections of Race, Food, and Development in West Papua." *The International Journal of Human Rights* 26, no. 5: 811–32.

Chatterjee, Upamanyu. 2018. *English, August: An Indian Story*. London: Faber and Faber.

Chettri, Mona. 2015. *Ethnicity and Democracy in the Eastern Himalayan Borderland*. Amsterdam: University of Amsterdam Press.

Chidester, David. 2001. *Christianity: A Global History*. New York: HarperCollins.

Chingarande, Dominica, Prosper Matondi, Gift Mungano, Godfrey Chagwiza, and Mabel Hungwe. 2020. "Zimbabwe Food Security Desk Research: Manicaland Province." Washington, DC: Research Technical Assistance Center. 1596 (2020): 32190. https://www.rtachesn.org/wp-content/uploads/2020/01/RTAC_Manicaland-Food-Security-Desk-Review_FINAL-3.pdf.

Chitando, E., and L. Togarasei. 2010. "'June 2008, verse 27': The Church and the 2008 Zimbabwean political crisis." *African Identities*, 8(2): 151–62.

Chomsky, Aviva, Barry Carr, Alfredo Prieto, and Pamela María Smorkaloff. 2019. *The Cuba Reader: History, Culture, Politics*, 2nd ed. Durham, NC: Duke University Press.

Clastres, Pierre. (1974) 2004. *A sociedade contra o estado*. Coletivo Sabotagem.

Clem, Julia, and Brandon Barthel. 2021. "A Look at Plant-Based Diets." *Missouri Medicine* 118, no. 3: 233–38.

Cock, Jacklyn. 2018. *Writing the Ancestral River: A Biography of the Kowie*. Johannesburg: Wits University Press.

Colás, Alejandro, Daniel Monterescu, and Ronald Ranta. 2022. "Introduction." In *'Going Native?' Settler Colonialism and Food*. Edited by Ronald Ranta, Alejandro Colás, and Daniel Monterescu, Cham, CHE: Palgrave Macmillan.

Collier, Gordon, and Ulrich Fleischmann. 2003. *A Pepper-Pot of Cultures: Aspects of Creolization in the Caribbean*. Amsterdam, NLD: Rodopi.

Colwell-Chanthaphonh, C. 2005. "When History Is Myth: Genocide and the Transmogrification of American Indians." *American Indian Culture and Research Journal*, 29 (2): 113–118.

Crasnow, S. 2021. "Feminist Science Studies: Reasoning from Cases." In *Making the Case: Feminist and Critical Race Philosophers Engage Case Studies*. Edited by H. E. Grasswick and N. A. McHugh. SUNY Press.

Crenshaw, Kimberlé. 1989. "Demarginalizing the Intersection of Race and Sex: A Black Feminist Critique of Antidiscrimination Doctrine, Feminist Theory and Antiracist Politics." *University of Chicago Legal Forum* vol. 1989, article 8.

Cruvinel, Régis Pereira, Luzia Regina Pereira Cruvinel, and Larissa Isaura Gomes. 2022. "Histórico de anomalias em saúde física e mental em trabalhadores do agronegócio na gestão de pessoas." *Research, Society and Development* 11, no. 7 (May 24): 1–8.

Cummings, Kate. 2019. "You Belong to the Land: A Conversation with Karen Washington and Leah Penniman." *Minding Nature* 13, no. 3 (Fall): 79-85.

Cunningham, Clark E. 1958. *The Postwar Migration of the Toba-Bataks to East Sumatra*. New Haven, CT: Yale University Southeast Asia Studies.

Dai, J. D., J. L. Yellowtail, A. Munoz-Salgado, J. J. Lopez, E. Ward-Griffin, C. E. Hawk, J. LeBlanc, N. Santos, A. Farero, A. E. Eason, and S. A. Fryberg. 2023. We Are Still Here: Omission and Perceived Discrimination Galvanized Civic Engagement Among Native Americans. *Psychological Science*, 34 (7): 739–753.

Daniel, Monodeep. 2019. *Society in India: Ambedkar's Vision, Essays from Christian Perspective.* Indian Society for Promoting Christian Knowledge.

De La Torre, Miguel A. 2002. *The Quest for the Cuban Christ: A Historical Search.* Gainesville: University Press of Florida.

________. 2022. "Towards an Ethics Para Joder: Decolonizing Minds by Transgressing Academic Borders." In *Resisting Occupation: A Global Struggle for Liberation.* Edited by Miguel A. De La Torre and Mitri Raheb. Lanham, MD: Lexington Books/Fortress Academic.

________. 2024. "What Do You Do When the God of Liberation Fails to Liberate?" In *Stirring Up Liberation Theologies.* Edited by Jione Havea. London: SCM.

de la Torre, Renée, and Martín Eloisa. 2016. "Religious Studies in Latin America." *Annual Review of Sociology* 42, no. 1: 473–92.

de las Casas, Bartolomé. (1561) 1971. *History of the Indies.* Unfinished. Edited and translated by Andree Collard. New York: Harper & Row.

Dena, Lal. n.d. "The First Mission that Sponsored William Pettigrew." In *Rev. William Pettigrew's Mission Reports and Letters 1891–1932.* Compiled and Reproduced by Reverend Champhang Jajo. Printed at Chandan Press, Santipur, Guwahati.

de Quesada, Gonzalo. 1925. *The Chinese & Cuban Independence.* Leipzig, Deutschland: Breitkopf & Hartel.

Desai, Kiran. 1998. *Hullaballoo in the Guava Orchard.* London: Faber and Faber.

de St. Dalmas, Henry Gershom Emeric. (1894) n.d. "Letter to Rev. C. Rudge, January 6, 1894." In *Rev. William Pettigrew's Mission Reports and Letters 1891–1932.* Compiled and Reproduced by Reverend Champhang Jajo. Printed at Chandan Press, Santipur, Guwahati.

Dolhare, María Itatí, and Sol Rojas-Lizana. 2017. "The Indigenous Concept of Vivir Bien in the Bolivian Legal Field: A Decolonial Proposal." *The Australian Journal of Indigenous Education* 47, no. 1: 19–29.

Downs. Frederick S. 1971. *The Mighty Works of God: A Brief History of the Council of Baptist Churches in North East India: The Mission Period 1836–1950.* Gauhati, Assam: Christian Literature Centre.

Drew, Georgina. 2021. "Coca-Cola and the Moral Economy of Rural Development in India." *South Asia: Journal of South Asian Studies* 44, no. 3 (June 2): 477–97.

Dube-Matutu, S. 2020. Farmers to get hay for livestock. *Chronicle*, July 7. https://www.chronicle.co.zw/farmers-to-get-hay-for-livestock/.

DuFord, Darrin. 2012. "Journey by Bottle: Uncovering the Allure of Guyanese Cassareep." *Gastronomica*, 12 (4): 27–30.

Dunford, Robin. 2017. "Toward a Decolonial Global Ethics." *Journal of Global Ethics* 13, no. 3: 380–97.

Dunham, Delicia. 2020. "On being Black and Vegan." In *Sistah Vegan: Black Women Speak on Food, Identity, Health, and Society*. Edited by A. Breeze Harper. New York: Lantern Books.

Earle, Rebecca 2012. *The Body of the Conquistador: Food, Race and the Colonial Experience in Spanish America, 1492–1700*. Cambridge: Cambridge University Press.

Easthope, A. 1998. Bhabha, hybridity and identity. *Textual Practice*, 12 (2): 341–48.

Eaton, Richard M. 1984. "Conversion to Christianity among the Nagas, 1876–1971." *The Indian Economic and Social History Review* 21, no. 1: 1–44.

"Ecuador: Annual Country Report." 2017–2022. *United Nations World Food Program*. Country Strategic Plan (2017–2022): 1–65.

Edwards, W., and K. Gibson. 1979. "An Ethnohistory of Amerindians in Guyana." *Ethnohistory* 26, no. 2: 161–75.

Egloff, Keith T. 1994. *First People: The Early Indians of Virginia*. Charlottesville: University Press of Virginia.

Ekström, Joel. 2020. *Food as a Weapon in Yemen: The Targeting of Food Security in a New War*. Batchelor Degree Thesis in Political Science. Lund, SWE: Lund University.

Eltis, D. 2021. Slave Voyages. https://www.slavevoyages.org/.

Ewbank, A. n.d. *This Sauce Can Allegedly Make a Stew Last a Lifetime*. Atlas Obscura. https://www.atlasobscura.com/foods/cassareep-sauce-pepperpot.

Fanon, Frantz. 1966. *The Wretched of the Earth*. Translated by Constance Farrington. New York: Evergreen.

Federici, Silvia. 2017. *Calibã e a Bruxa: Mulheres, Corpos e Acumulação Primitiva*. São Paulo: Editora Elefante.

Fehskens, Erin M. 2013. "Desai's Hullaballoo in the Guava Orchard as Global Literature." *CLCWeb: Comparative Literature and Culture* 15, no. 6: 1–10.

Femenías, María Luisa. 2020. "From Women's Movements to Feminist Theories (and Vice Versa)." In *Theories of the Flesh: Latinx and Latin American Feminisms, Transformation, and Resistance*. Edited by Andrea J. Pitts, Mariana Ortega, and José Medina. New York: Oxford University Press.

Ferguson, Niall. 2021. *Doom: The Politics of Catastrophe*. New York: Penguin Press.

Figueroa-Vásquez, Y. C. 2020. *Decolonizing Diasporas: Radical Mappings of Afro-Atlantic Literature*. Northwestern University Press.

Finch, W. A. 1990. The Immigration Reform and Control Act of 1986: A Preliminary Assessment. *Social Service Review*, 64 (2): 244–260.

Fisher, Andy. 2019. "Ecopsychology as Decolonial Praxis." *Ecopsychology* 11, no. 3: 145–55.

Fisk, Ernest K. 1966. *New Guinea on the Threshold: Aspects of Social, Political, and Economical Development*. Canberra: Australia National University Press.

Foley, Neil. 2014. *Mexicans in the Making of America*. Cambridge, MA: Belknap Press of Harvard University Press.

Food and Agriculture Organization of the United Nations (FAO). 2006. *Food security*. Policy Brief 2. http://www.fao.org/fileadmin/templates/faoitaly/documents/pdf/pdf_Food_Security_Cocept_Note.pdf.

________. 2022. *Meat Market Review: Emerging trends and outlook*. Rome: Food and Agriculture Organization of the United Nations.

Fuller, Camphor J. 2004. *The Camphor Flame: Popular Hinduism and Society in India*. Princeton: Princeton University Press.

Furer-Haimendorf, Christoph von. 1939. *The Naked Nagas*. London: Methuen & Co.

Ganti, Tejaswini. 2014. "Neoliberalism." *Annual Review of Anthropology* 43: 89–104.

Garcia-Weyandt, Cydny. 2023. "Teachings of Tatéi Niwetsika: Native Maize from Northern Mexico." In *New Prospects of Maize*. Edited by Prashant Kaushik. London, UK: IntechOpen.

Gardinier, David. 1968. "Decolonization." In *Handbook of World History: Concepts and Issues*. Edited by Joseph Dunner. 268–72. London: Owen.

Garth, Hanna. 2013. *Food and Identity in the Caribbean*. London: Bloomsbury Academic.

George, Cherian. 2020. *Air-Conditioned Nation Revisited: Essays on Singapore Politics*. Singapore: Ethos Books.

Gold, Amanda, Wenson Fung, Susan Gabbard, and Daniel Carroll. 2022. *Findings from the National Agricultural Workers Survey (NAWS) 2019–2020: A Demographic and Employment Profile of United States Farmworkers*. Washington D.C.: U.S. Department of Labor.

Gomberg, Paul. 2017. "Workers Without Rights." *Symposion: Theoretical and Applied Inquiries in Philosophy and Social Sciences* 4, no. 1: 49–76.

Gómez, Laura E. 2008. *Manifest Destinies: The Making of the Mexican American Race*. New York: New York University Press.

Gómez-Barris, M. 2017. *The Extractive Zone: Social Ecologies and Decolonial Perspectives*. Duke University Press.

González, Suzy. 2021. "Staying Afloat." *Ofrenda Magazine* Issue 4 (September): 44–49.

Gracia, Jorge J. E. 2007. *Race or Ethnicity?: On Black and Latino Identity*. Ithaca, NY: Cornell University Press.

Gratton, Brian, and Emily Klancher Merchant. 2016. "La Raza : Mexicans in the United States Census." *Journal of Policy History* 28, no. 4 (October): 537–67.

Guanche, Jesús. 1983. *Procesos etnoculturales de Cuba*. La Habana: Editorial Letras Cubanas.

Hanke, Steve H., and Alex K. Kwok. 2009. "On the Measurement of Zimbabwe's Hyperinflation." *Cato Journal* 29: 353–64.

Harding, Vincent. 1981. *There Is a River: The Black Struggle for Freedom in America*. New York: Harcourt Brace Jovanovich.

Hardwick, Louise. 2014. "Creolizing the Caribbean 'Coolie': A Biopolitical Reading of Indian Indentured Labourers and the Ethnoclass Hierarchy." *International Journal of Francophone Studies* 17, no. 3: 397–419.

Hargreaves, John D. 1996. *Decolonization in Africa*. Second edition. London: Longman.

Harper, A. Breeze. 2020. *Sistah Vegan: Black Female Vegans Speak on Food, Identity, Health, and Society*. New York: Lantern Books.

________. 2011. "Vegans of Color, Racialized Embodiment, and Problematics of the "Exotic." In *Cultivating Food Justice: Race, Class, and Sustainability*. Edited by Alison Hope Alkon. Cambridge: MIT Press.

Harris, Melanie. 2017. *Ecowomanism: African American Women and Earth-Honoring Faiths*. New York: Orbis Books.

Havea, Jione. Forthcoming in 2024. "Moana economies: A theological invitation." In *Unsettling Theologies: Memory, Identity, and Place*. Edited by Brian F. Kolia and Michael Mawson. London: Palgrave.

________. Forthcoming. "Moana criticisms: Recollecting biblical studies in Pasifika." *Samoa Journal of Theology* 3.

________. 2003. *Elusions of Control: Biblical Law on the Words of Women*. Atlanta: Society of Biblical Literature.

________. 2018. *Sea of Readings: The Bible in the South Pacific*. Atlanta: Society of Biblical Literature.

________. 2021a. "The Authors/Interpreters, a Twig, and Paradise: In the Shadows of Maratja Dhamarrandji, Emmanuel Garibay, and Mariana Waqa." *The Bible and Critical Theory* 17 no. 1: 82–89.

________. 2021b. "Going Native: ReStorying Theology and Hermeneutics." *Modern Believing* 62 no. 4: 349–57.

________. 2021c. *Jonah: An Earth Bible Commentary*. London: Bloomsbury.

________. 2021d. Losing Ground: Reading Ruth in the Pacific. London: SCM.

Havea, Jione, Margaret Aymer, and Steed Vernyl Davidson, eds. 2015. *Islands, Islanders, and the Bible: RumInations*. Atlanta: Society of Biblical Literature.

Havea, Jione, and Peter H. W. Lau, eds. 2020. *Reading Ecclesiastes from Asia and Pasifika*. Atlanta: Society of Biblical Literature.

Havea, Jione, David J. Neville, and Elaine M. Wainwright, eds. 2014. *Bible, Borders, Belonging(s): Engaging Readings from Oceania*. Atlanta: Society of Biblical Literature.

Henderson, Thomas Paul. 2017. "State-Peasant Movement Relations and the Politics of Food Sovereignty in Mexico and Ecuador." *Journal of Peasant Studies* 44, no. 1: 33–35.

Henry, D. E. 2019. *More Than 50 Years Since Independence, Colonial Violence Plagues Guyana and Its Diaspora*. Pulitzer Center. https://pulitzercenter.org/stories/more-50-years-independence-colonial-violence-plagues-guyana-and-its-diaspora.

Hernández, K. L. 2006. "The Crimes and Consequences of Illegal Immigration: A Cross-Border Examination of Operation Wetback, 1943 to 1954." *The Western Historical Quarterly*, 37(4): 421. https://doi.org/10.2307/25443415.

Higman, B. W. 2012. *How Food Made History*. Oxford, UK: Wiley-Blackwell.

Hirshberg, Dan. 2016. *Remembering the Lotus-Born*. Somerville, MA: Wisdom Publications.

Holmes, Seth. 2013. *Fresh Fruit, Broken Bodies: Migrant Farmworkers in the United States*. University of California Press.

Horam, Mashangthei. 1977. *Social and Cultural Life of Nagas*. Delhi: P.R. Publishing.

Horam, Ringkahao. 2013. *The Tangkhul Folk Poetry in Song* (Haolaa). Imphal, Manipur: Mr & Mrs. Dr. R. Horam and NCDS.

Horst, Megan, and Amy Marion. 2019. "Racial, Ethnic and Gender Inequities in Farmland Ownership and Farming in the U.S." *Agriculture and Human Values* 36, no. 2 (March): 1–16.

Hoskins, Christopher M. 2023. "Rebuilding Together Through Buen Vivir: Democratic Collectives and Ecuadorian Liberation Theologies in the Face of the IMF and Disaster Capitalism." *Journal of Pastoral Theology* 1, no. 1: 1–18.

Houston, Lynn Marie. 2005. *Food Culture in the Caribbean*. Greenwood Press.

Hoyos, Héctor. 2019. *Things with a History: Transcultural Materialism and the Literature of Extraction in Contemporary Latin America*. New York: Columbia University Press.

Hughes, Robert G. 2003. *Diet, Food Supply and Obesity in the Pacific*. Geneva, CHE: World Health Organization.

Hughes, Robert G., and Mark A. Lawrence. 2005. "Globalisations, Food and Health in Pacific Island Countries." *Asia Pacific Journal of Clinical Nutrition* 14 no. 4: 298–306.

Hungwe, E., J. Masaka, V. Makuvaro, and E. Tombo. 2020. "Increased Sorghum (Sorghum bicolor, L) Productivity: Unlocking its potential for food crisis mitigation for small holder communal farmers in the Semi-Arid regions: A case of the Zambezi Valley Region in Zimbabwe." *International Journal of Agriculture, Biology & Environment* 1, no. 03 (2020): 01–14.

Hutasoit, Resmi, Izak M. Lattu, and Ebenhaizer I Nuban Timo. 2020. "Kekuatan Simbolik Beras Dalam Ritus Kehidupan Masyarakat Batak

Toba." *Anthropos: Jurnal Antropologi Sosial Dan Budaya* 5, no. 2 (January 6): 183–95.

Hyatt, V. L., R. M. Nettleford, and S. Institution. 1995. *Race Discourse Origin Amer*. Smithsonian.

Idrovo, C., J. Grant, and J. R. Yanoff. 2022. *Discovery of Oil Could Bring Migrant Labor Opportunities and Climate Displacement Challenges for Guyana*. Migrationpolicy.org. July 26, 2022. https://www.migrationpolicy.org/article/guyana-discovery-oil-labor-migration-climate-displacement.

Irons, Dylan Alexander. 2022. *The Political Economy of Forced Migration: How Weaponized Poverty Leads to Displacement*. Doctoral dissertation. Nashville: Vanderbilt University.

Ishmael, Odeen. 2013. *The Guyana Story: From Earliest Times to Independence*. Bloomington, IN: Xlibris Corporation.

Jeyaseelan, Lazar. 1996. *Impact of the Missionary Movement in Manipur*. New Delhi: Scholar Publishing.

Junior, Marco Antonio Mitidiero, and Yamila Goldfarb. 2021. *O agro não é tech, o agro não é pop e muito menos tudo*. São Paulo: Friedrich-Ebert-Stifung.

Kaldor, Mary. 2012. *New and Old Wars: Organized Violence in a Global Era*. New York: Polity Press.

Kannuri, Nanda Kishore, and Sushrut Jadhav. 2021. "Cultivating Distress: Cotton, Caste, and Farmer Suicides in India." *Anthropology & Medicine* 28, no. 4: 558–75.

Keuning, Johannes. 1958. *The Toba Batak, Formerly and Now*. Translated by Claire Holt. Ithaca: Cornell University Press.

Kharay, Woryaomi. 2021. "Christianity and the 'Others': On Conversion of the Tangkhul Nagas." *Journal of Religion and Society* 23: 1–21.

Kharingpam, A. C. 2020. "Revisiting Pettigrew's Education: The Ushering of the Colonial Ideology Through Schools and Textbooks Amongst the Tangkhul Nagas (1896–1938)." *Contemporary Literary Review India* 7, no. 3: 1–12.

Khongreiwo, Rammathot. 2011. "Landscapes and Pre-Christian Belief System: Cosmology, God, Spirits and 'Land of the Dead'." *Journal of Tribal Studies* 16, no. 1: 43–67.

Kikon, Dolly. 2021. "Bamboo Shoot in Our Blood: Fermenting Flavors and Identities in Northeast India." *Current Anthropology* 62, no. 24: S376–87.

Kikon, Dolly, and Bengt Karlsson. 2019. *Leaving the Land*. Cambridge: Cambridge University Press.

Kimmerer, Robin Wall. 2013. *Braiding Sweetgrass: Indigenous Wisdom, Scientific Knowledge, and the Teachings of Plants*. Minneapolis: Milkweed Editions.

Ko, Aph. 2019. *Racism as Zoological Witchcraft: A Guide to Getting Out*. New York: Lantern Books.

Ko, Aph, and Syl Ko. 2017. *Aphro-ism: Essays on Pop Culture, Feminism, and Black Veganism from Two Sisters*. New York: Lantern Books.

Kolia, Brian F. Forthcoming. *Carrying Qohelet's Maota (House): An Australia-Samoan Diasporic Reading of Wisdom in Ecclesiastes*. Atlanta: Society of Biblical Literature.

Konghay, Ikrormi. 2016. *The Tangkhul Naga Community of Past, Present and Future*. Imphal, Manipur: Development of Human Potential.

Kozok, Uli. 1991. "The Economic Foundation of the Society." In *The Batak*. New York: Thames and Hudson.

________. 2010. *Utusan Damai Di Kemelut Perang: Peran Zending Dalam Perang Toba Berdasarkan Laporan I. L. Nommensen Dan Penginjil RMG Lain*. Jakarta, IDN: Yayasan Pustaka Obor Indonesia.

Krenak, Ailton. 2019. *Ideias para adiar o fim do mundo*. São Paulo: Companhia das Letras.

KSPPM, Tim. 2021. *Mangan Sian Tano Ni Ompung: Food Estate versus Kedaulatan Petani*. Yogyakarta, IDN: INSISTPress.

Kumar, A. 2017. *Coolies of the Empire: Indentured Indians in the Sugar Colonies, 1830–1920* (1st ed.). University Press.

Kumar, Sangeet. 2010. *Postcolonial Identity in a Globalizing India: Case Studies in Visual, Musical and Oral Culture*. PhD Dissertation. University of Iowa, July 2010.

LaBennett, O. 2024. *Global Guyana: Shaping Race, Gender, and Environment in the Caribbean and Beyond*. New York: NYU Press.

Leff, Enrique. 2012. "Pensamiento Ambiental Latinoamericano: Patrimonio de un Saber para la Sustentabilidad." *Environmental Ethics* 34, no. 1 (Winter): 97–112.

Legassick, Martin. 2010. *The Struggle for the Eastern Cape 1800–1854: Subjugation and the Roots of South African Democracy*. Johannesburg: KMM Review.

Leong, N. 2012. *Racial Capitalism* (SSRN Scholarly Paper 2009877). https://doi.org/10.2139/ssrn.2009877.

Lepcha, Charisma K. 2021. "Lepcha Water View and Climate Change in Sikkim Himalaya." In *Environmental Humanities in the New Himalayas*. Edited by Dan Smyer Yu and Erik de Maaker. New York: Routledge.

Li, Tania, and Pujo Semedi. *Plantation Life: Corporate Occupation in Indonesia's Oil Palm Zone*. Durham: Duke University Press, 2021.

Lionnet, Françoise, Shu-mei Shih, Étienne Balibar, Dominique Chancé, Pheng Cheah, Leo Ching, Barnor Hesse, and Anne Donadey. 2011. *The Creolization of Theory*, Durham: Duke University Press.

Lipsitz, G. 2007. The Racialization of Space and the Spatialization of Race: Theorizing the Hidden Architecture of Landscape. *Landscape Journal*, 26 (1): 10–23.

Longkumer, Arkotong. 2016. "Rice-Beer, Purification and Debates over Religion and Culture in Northeast India." In *South Asia: Journal of South Asian Studies*, 39.2 (2016): 1–18.

Lugones, María. 2020. "Revisiting Gender: A Decolonial Approach." In *Theories of the Flesh: Latinx and Latin American Feminisms, Transformation, and Resistance*. Edited by Andrea J. Pitts, Mariana Ortega, and José Medina. New York: Oxford University.

Luikham, Thisan. 1948. *A Short History of the Manipur Baptist Christian: Golden Jubilee (in Tangkhul)*. Ukhrul, Manipur: N.E. Christian Association.

Lungleng, Phongreingam. 2011. *Tangkhul Festivals, Rituals and Sacrifices*. Ukhrul, Manipur: TTA.

Macarena Gomez-Barris. 2017. *The Extractive Zone: Social Ecologies and Decolonial Perspectives*. Durham, NC: Duke University Press.

Macinnis, Peter. 2002. *Bittersweet: The Story of Sugar*. Crows Nest, Australia: Allen & Unwin.

Madimu, T., 2020. Food imports, hunger and state making in Zimbabwe, 2000–2009. *Journal of Asian and African Studies*, 55(1): 128–44.

Maddock, R. T., 1978. The economic and political characteristics of food as a diplomatic weapon. *Journal of Agricultural Economics*, 29(1): 31–41.

Mailo, Mosese. 2016. *Bible-ing my Samoan*. Apia: Piula.

Makonye, F. 2021. The Inherent Resort to Violence in Opposition Politics: A Synthesis of the Post-2005 Movement for Democratic Change (MDC) Formations in Zimbabwe. *African Journal of Peace and Conflict Studies*, 10(1): 77–99.

Maldonado-Torres, Nelson. 2007. "On the Coloniality of Being: Contributions to the Development of a Concept." *Cultural Studies* 21, no. 2–3 (March): 240–70.

Mandavilli, Sujay R. 2019. *Articulating Comprehensive Frameworks on Socio-Cultural Change: Social and Cultural Change in Twenty-First Century Anthropology*. Chennai: Notion Press.

Mann, Barbara Alice. 2005. *George Washington's War on Native America*. Westport, CT: Greenwood.

Manse, Maarten. 2022. "Two Sides of the Same Coin: Direct Taxation and Negotiated Governance in Colonial Indonesia." *Journal of Social History* 56, no. 2 (December 2, 2022): 411–38. https://doi.org/10.1093/jsh/shac050.

Marín-Dale, Margarita. 2016. *Decoding Andean Mythology*. Salt Lake City: University of Utah.

Marte, L. 2013. Versions of Dominican Mangú: Intersections of Gender and Nation in Caribbean Self-making. In H. Garth, ed., *Food and Identity in the Caribbean*. Bloomsbury Academic.

Martínez Novo, Carmen. 2018. "Ventriloquism, Racism, and the Politics of Decoloniality in Ecuador." *Cultural Studies* 32, no. 3: 389–413.

McCartney, Martha. 2000. *Jamestown Island Volume 1: Narrative History*. Williamsburg, VA: U.S. Department of the Interior.

McKay, Ben, Ryan Nehring, and Marygold Walsh-Dilley. 2014. "The 'State' of Food Sovereignty in Latin America: Political Projects and Alternative Pathways in Venezuela, Ecuador, and Bolivia." *Journal of Peasant Studies* 41, no. 6: 1175–1200.

McLennan, Amy K., and Stanley J. Ulijaszek. 2015. "Obesity Emergence in the Pacific Islands: Why Understanding Colonial History and Social Change Is Important." In *Public Health Nutrition Vol 18*. Edited by Charlotte Evans. New York: Cambridge University Press.

Memmi, Albert. 2021. *The Albert Memmi Reader*. Edited by Jonathan Judaken and Michael Lejman. Lincoln: University of Nebraska Press.

Méndez, Michael, Genevieve Flores-Haro, and Lucas Zucker. 2020. "The (In) Visible Victims of Disaster: Understanding the Vulnerability of Undocumented Latino/a and Indigenous Immigrants." *Geoforum* 116 (November): 50–62.

Mercado, Geovana, and Carsten Nico Hjortsø. 2023. "Explaining the Development Policy Implementation Gap: A Case of a Failed Food Sovereignty Policy in Bolivia." *World Development* 166, no. 106216: 1–15.

Messer, Ellen. 1991. *Food Wars: Hunger as a Weapon of War in 1994*. Providence, RI: Alan Shawn Feinstein World Hunger Program, Brown University.

________. 1998. "Conflict as a Cause of Hunger." In *Who's Hungry? And How Do We Know?: Food Shortage, Poverty, and Deprivation.* Edited by Laurie Fields DeRose, Ellen Messer, and Sara Millman. Tokyo: United Nations University Press.

Mignolo, Walter D. 2000. *Local Histories/Global Designs: Coloniality, Subaltern Knowledges, and Border Thinking*. Princeton: Princeton University Press.

________. 2020. "On Decoloniality: Second Thoughts." *Postcolonial Studies* 23, no. 4: 612–18.

Miller, Daniel. 2005. "Coca-Cola: A Black Sweet Drink from Trinidad." In *The Cultural Politics of Food and Eating: A Reader*. Edited by James L. Watson and Melissa L. Caldwell. Hoboken, NJ: Blackwell Publishing.

Mintz, Sidney W. 1986. *Sweetness and Power: The Place of Sugar in Modern History*. New York: Penguin.

Misir, Prem. 2010. *Racial Ethnic Imbalance in Guyana Public Bureaucracies: The Tension between Exclusion and Representation*, 1st edition. Lewiston, NY: Edwin Mellen Press.

Mistry, Rohinton. 1995. *A Fine Balance*. London: Faber and Faber.

Mize, Ronald L., and Alicia C. S. Swords. 2010. *Consuming Mexican Labor: From the Bracero Program to NAFTA*. Toronto: University of Toronto Press.

Mlambo, A. S. 2017. From an industrial powerhouse to a nation of vendors: Over two decades of economic decline and deindustrialization in Zimbabwe 1990–2015. *Journal of Developing Societies*, 33(1): 99–125.

Moe-Lobeda, Cyntha. 2020. "Christ's Love in the Midst of Pandemic: Moving the World Toward an Economy of Life." *The Ecumenical Review* 72, no. 4 (October): 553–68.

Molina, N. 2014. *How Race Is Made in America: Immigration, Citizenship, and the Historical Power of Racial scripts*. University of California Press.

Monodeep, Daniel. 2019. Society in India: Ambedkar's Vision, Essays from Christian Perspective. Indian Society for Promoting Christian Knowledge.

Montejano, D. 1987. *Anglos and Mexicans in the Making of Texas, 1836–1986* (1st ed.). University of Texas Press.

Montejo, Esteban. 1968. *The Autobiography of a Runaway Slave*. Edited by Miguel Barnet. Translated by Jocasta Innes. New York: Pantheon Books.

Moore, P. H., F. P. Haggard, and C. E. Burdette. 1895. "William Pettigrew at Sibsagar Conference (1895)." In *The Assam Mission of the American Baptist Missionary Union: Minutes, Resolutions, and Historical Reports of the Fourth Triennial Conference Held in Sibsagar, December 14–22, 1895* (Calcutta, India: Baptist Mission Press).

Moyo, Philani. 2022. "The Political Economy of Zimbabwe's Food Crisis, 2019–2020." *Journal of Asian and African Studies* (August 26, 2022): 1–16.

Mpofu, T. 2019. Drought claims more than 10,000 cattle in Zimbabwe. *Farmers Weekly*. November 5. https://www.farmersweekly.co.za/agri-news/africa/drought-claims-more-than-10-000-cattle-in-zimbabwe/.

Mudzonga, Evangelista, and Tendai Chigwada. 2009. "A Case Study of Zimbabwe's Food Security Winnipeg, MB: International Institute for Sustainable Development.

Murray-Li, Tania, and Pujo Semedi. 2021. *Plantation Life: Corporate Occupation in Indonesia's Oil Palm Zone*. Durham: Duke University Press.

Muttoo, H. 1999. From Multiculturalism to Culturalism. *Caribbean Quarterly* 45 (2–3): 109–113.

Nail, Thomas. 2018. *Being and Motion*. New York: Oxford University Press.

Nasr, Seyyed Hossien. 1997. *Man and Nature: The Spiritual Crisis in Modern Man*. Chicago: ABC International Group.

National Agricultural Statistics Service. 2017. Census volume 1, chapter 2: State level data. Table 7: Hired farm labor—Workers and payroll:

2017. U.S. Department of Agriculture. https://www.nass.usda.gov/Publications/AgCensus/2017/Full_Report/Volume_1,_Chapter_2_US_State_Level/st99_2_0007_0007.pdf.

Needham, Joseph. 1996. *Science and Civilization in China*. Cambridge: Cambridge University Press.

Nelson, Cynthia. 2010. *Tastes Like Home: My Caribbean Cookbook*, 1st edition. Kingston, JAM: Ian Randle.

Newton, M. J. 2014. "The Race Leapt at Sauteurs": Genocide, Narrative, and Indigenous Exile from the Caribbean Archipelago. *Caribbean Quarterly* 60 (2): 5–28.

Ngakang, Tuisem. 2022. "Evangelizing the Nagas in the Second Half of the Nineteenth and First Half of the Twentieth Century: Missionary Encounter and Cultural Disarming." In *Tribe, Space and Mobilisation Colonial Dynamics and Post-Colonial Dilemma in Tribal Studies*. Edited by Maguni Charan Behera. Singapore: Springe.

Nofoaiga, Vaitusi. 2017. *A Samoan Reading of Discipleship in Matthew 8*. Atlanta: Society of Biblical Literature.

Omi, M., and H. Winant. 2015. *Racial Formation in the United States* (3rd ed.). Routledge/Taylor & Francis Group.

On, Bat-Ami Bar. 2012. "War and Food." In *Encyclopedia of Food and Agricultural Ethics*, 2nd edition. Edited by David M. Kaplan. New York: Springer: 2455–61

Ortiz, Fernando. (1940a) 1963. *Contrapunteo cubano del tabaco y el azúcar*. La Habana: Dirección de Publicaciones Universidad Central de Las Villas.

________. 1940b. *Los factores humanos de la cubanidad*. La Habana: Revista Bimestre Cubana, XLV.

________. 1947. *Cuban Counterpoint; Tobacco and Sugar*. Translated by Harriet De Onis. New York: Alfred A. Knopf.

Ortiz, Paul. 2018. *An African American and Latinx History of the United States*. Boston: Beacon Press.

Padilla-Meléndez, Antonio, et al. 2022. "Understanding the Entrepreneurial Resilience of Indigenous Women Entrepreneurs as a Dynamic Process: The Case of Quechuas in Bolivia." *Entrepreneurship and Regional Development* 34, no. 9–10: 852–67.

Padula, Raphael, Matheus de Freitas Cecílio, Igor Candido de Oliveira, and Caio Jorge Prado. 2023. "Guyana: Oil, Internal Disputes, the USA and Venezuela." *Contexto Internacional* 45, no. 1: 1–25.

Page, Sam L. J., and Helán E. Page. 1991. Western Hegemony over African Agriculture in Southern Rhodesia and Its Continuing Threat to Food Security in Independent Zimbabwe. *Agriculture and Human Values* 8: 3–18.

Pedersen, Paul Bodholdt. 1970. *Batak Blood and Protestant Soul: The Development of National Batak Churches in North Sumatra*. Grand Rapids, MI: William B. Eerdmans.

Pelzer, Karl. 1978. *Planter and Peasant: Colonial Policy and the Agrarian Struggle in East Sumatera 1863–1947*. Leiden, UK: Brill.

Peña, Karla. 2013. "Institutionalizing Food Sovereignty in Ecuador." *Food Sovereignty: A Critical Dialogue*. International Conference Yale University. (September 14–15, 2013): 1–25.

Pettigrew, William. (1894) n.d. "Manipur, The Bond: May 1894." In *Rev. William Pettigrew's Mission Reports and Letters 1891–1932*. Compiled and Reproduced by Reverend Champhang Jajo. Printed at Chandan Press, Santipur, Guwahati.

________. 1897a. "Ukhrul—1896," *The Baptist Missionary Magazine* 77 no. 7 (January): 325–26.

________. 1897b. "The Beginning of Ukhrul Station (1897)." *Baptist Missionary Magazine* 77, no. 9 (September): 526.

________. 1899. "Report from the Tangkhul Naga Field." In *The Assam of the American Baptist Foreign Mission Society: Minutes, Resolutions and Historical of the Fifth Triennial Conference, February 11–19, 1899*. Calcutta: The Baptist Mission Press.

________. 1909. "Kathe Kasham: The 'Soul Departure' Feast as Practised by the Tangkhul Nagas, Manipur, Assam." *Journal of Proceedings of the Asiatic Society of Bengal* vol. V: 37–46.

________. 1986. *Forty Years in Manipur Assam: Mission Reports of Rev. William Pettigrew*. Compiled by Jonah M. Solo and K. Mahangthei. Imphal, Manipur: Mrs. M. Asenath and Mrs. K. Ruth.

Pilcher, Jeffrey M., ed. 2012. *The Oxford Handbook of Food History*. New York: Oxford University Press.

Pompeia, Caio. 2021. *Formação política do agronegócio*. São Paulo: Editora Elefante.

Pope Francis. 2015. *Laudato Si': On Care for Our Common Home*. Vatican.

Pope Paul VI. 1965. *Gaudium et Spes*. Vatican Council II, December 1965.

Poulan, Michael. 2006. *Omnivore's Dilemma: A Natural History of Four Meals*. New York: Penguin.

Preston, Jen. 2017. "Racial Extractivism and White Settler Colonialism: An Examination of the Canadian Tar Sands Mega-Projects." *Cultural Studies* 31, no. 2–3 (May 4): 353–75.

Purba, O. H. S., and Elvis F. Purba. 1997. *Migrasi Spontan Batak Toba (Marserak): Sebab, Motif Dan Akibat Perpindahan Penduduk Dari Dataran Tinggi Toba*. Medan, IDN: Monora.

Radcliffe, Sarah A. 2014. "Gendered Frontiers of Land Control: Indigenous Territory, Women, and Contests Over Land in Ecuador." *Gender, Place, and Culture* 21, no. 7: 854–71.

Ragui, Taimaya. 2023. "Decolonising Knowledge in the Tangkhul Naga Context." Paper presented at "From Colonial Modernity to Decolonisation: The British Empire and Beyond." University of Auckland. September 15–16, 2023.

Richards-Greaves, Gillian. 2013. "The Intersections of 'Guyanese Food' and Constructions of Gender, Race, and Nationhood." In *Food and Identity in the Caribbean*. Edited by Hanna Garth, 75–94. London; New York: Bloomsbury.

Rickford, J. R. 1987. *Dimensions of a Creole Continuum: History, Texts, and Linguistic Analysis of Guyanese Creole*. Stanford University Press.

Ritzer, George, and Elizabeth L. Malone. 2000. "Globalization Theory: Lessons from the Exportation of McDonaldization and the New Means of Consumption." American Studies (Lawrence) 41, no. 2/3: 97–118.

Ritzer, George, and ProQuest. 2006. *The Blackwell Companion to Globalization*. Oxford: Blackwell.

Rivera Cusicanqui, Silvia. 2010. *Ch'ixinakax utxiwa : una reflexión sobre prácticas y discursos descolonizadores*. Buenos Aires: Tinta Limón.

Robertson, Roland. 1992. *Globalization: Social Theory and Global Culture*. London: SAGE.

Robertson, R., and K. E. White. 2006. What is Globalization. In *The Blackwell Companion to Globalization*. Oxford: Blackwell.

Robinson, Cedric J. 2005. *Black Marxism: The Making of the Black Radical Tradition*. Chapel Hill: University of North Carolina Press.

Rodney, Walter. 2011. *How Europe Underdeveloped Africa*. Baltimore: Black Classic Press.

Rose, Asquith. 2023. "Support for President Ali's Policies and His 'One Guyana' Initiative Is Widespread." *Guyana Chronicle*, May 3, 2023, sec. Letters.

Rousseau, M., and S. Rousseau. 2018. *Provisions: The Roots of Caribbean Cooking—150 Vegetarian Recipes* (Illustrated edition). Da Capo Lifelong Books.

Roux, H. F. de. n.d. *Creolization in the Caribbean*. Smithsonian Folklife Festival. Retrieved March 8, 2024, from https://festival.si.edu/articles/1989/creolization-in-the-caribbean.

Runganga, R., W. Njoroge, and S. Mishi. 2022. Restoration of land acquired for resettlement and the fast-track land reform programme in Zimbabwe. *Sustainability*, 14(15): 9178.

Rusinamhodzi, L. 2015. Tinkering on the periphery: labour burden not crop productivity increased under no-till planting basins on smallholder farms in Murehwa district, Zimbabwe. *Field Crops Research*, 170, 66–75.

Said, Edward W. 1979. *Orientalism*. First paperback edition. New York: Vintage.

Salazar, Daniela. 2022. "The Constitutional History of Ecuador: Twenty Constitutions and Counting." In *The Oxford Handbook of Constitutional Law in Latin America*. Edited by Conrado Hübner Mendes, Roberto Gargarella, and Sebestián Guidi. New York: Oxford University.

Sanders, A. 1995. Protected Status and the Amerindians of Guyana: A Comparative Examiniation. *Social and Economic Studies* 44 (2/3): 125–141.

Schacht, R. N. 2013. Cassava and the Makushi: A Shared History of Resiliency and Transformation. In *Food and Identity in the Caribbean* (1–192). Bloomsbury Publishing. https://www.torrossa.com/en/resources/an/5204958.

Sen, Amartya. 2009. *The Idea of Justice*. Cambridge: Harvard University Press.

Sen, C. T. 2009. *Curry: A Global History*. London: Reaktion.

Shankar, Deepa. 2007. *What Is the Progress in Elementary Education Participation in India during the Last Two Decades?* New Delhi: Oxford University Press.

Sherman, D. George. 2020. *Rice, Rupees, and Ritual: Economy and Society among the Samosir Batak of Sumatra*. Stanford, CA: Stanford University Press.

Sherman, Sean, and Beth Dooley. 2017. *The Sioux Chef's Indigenous Kitchen*. Minneapolis: University of Minnesota Press.

Shimray, Y. K. n.d. "William Pettigrew and the Hill People." In *Rev. William Pettigrew's Mission Reports and Letters 1891–1932*. Compiled and reproduced by Reverend Champhang Jajo. Santipur, Guwahati: Chandan Press.

Shimrei, Console Zamreinao. 2016. "Livelihood Practices and Environmental Changes with Special Reference to Ukhrul District of Manipur." *Language in India* 16 no. 6: 43–56.

Siagian, Riris Johanna. 2016. *Sahala Bagi Pemimpin Dulu Dan Kini*. Pematangsiantar, IDN: Sekolah Tinggi Theologia HKBP6.

Siahaan, Manat, Lusia Rahajeng, Djoys Rantung, and Noh Ibrahim. 2022. "Peran Marsiadapari Dan Gugur Gunung Sebagai Landasan Dalam Teknologi Pendidikan Agama Kristen Di Sekolah." *Jurnal Educatio FKIP UNMA* 8, no. 3 (September 24): 1026–37.

Sibarani, Robert. 2018. "Batak Toba Society's Local Wisdom of Mutual Cooperation in Toba Lake Area: A Linguistic Anthropology Study." *International Journal of Human Rights in Health Care* 11, no. 1: 40–55.

Sibeth, Achim. 1991. *The Batak*. New York: Thames and Hudson.

Sihombing, Hesron H. 2023. "The Batak-Christian Theology of Land: Towards a Postcolonial Comparative Theology." *CrossCurrents* 73, no. 1 (March): 42–63.

Sina, Anjeza. 2018. "The Constitutional Protection of the Right to Food in Bolivia and Ecuador." In *Food Diversity Between Rights, Duties, and Autonomies: Legal Perspectives for a Scientific, Cultural, and Social Debate on the Right to Food and Agroecology*. Edited by Alessandro Isoni, Michele Troisi, and Maurizia Pierri. Cham: Springer International.

Sinaga, Anicetus B. 2014. *Allah Tinggi Batak-Toba*. Yogyakarta: Kanisius.

Sinclair, Donald, and Carolann Marcus. 2015. "Aboriginal Food: Traditional Dishes Surviving in the Fast Food Era." In *The Routledge Handbook of Sustainable Food and Gastronomy*. Routledge.

Singh, Darshan. 2009. "Development of Scheduled Castes in India—A Review." *Journal of Rural Development* 28, no. 4: 529–42.

Singh, Leiren. 1996. "Reverend William Pettigrew and Modern Education in Manipur." In *Rev. William Pettigrew: A Pioneer Missionary of Manipur*. Imphal, India: Fraternal Green Cross.

Smith, Linda Tuhiwai. 1999. *Decolonizing Methodologies: Research and Indigenous Peoples*. Zed Books.

Srivastava, Sonakshi. 2022. "On Reading Transformation in Desai's Hullaballoo in the Guava Orchard." *Spark*, 8: 1–13.

Stanley, Brian. 1998. "The Legacy of Robert Arthington." *International Bulletin of Missionary Research* 22, no. 4 (October): 166–71.

Staples, B. 2018. A Fate Worse Than Slavery, Unearthed in Sugar Land. *The New York Times*, October 27, 2018. https://www.nytimes.com/2018/10/27/opinion/sugar-land-texas-graves-slavery.html.

Stoler, Ann. 1985. "Perceptions of Protest: Defining the Dangerous in Colonial Sumatra." *American Ethnologist* 12, no. 4: 642–58.

Tamang, Jyoti Prakash. 2001. "Food Culture in the Eastern Himalayas," *Journal of Himalayan Research and Cultural Foundation* 5, no. 3–4: 107–18.

________. 2005. *Food Culture of Sikkim*. Gangtok, IND: Information and Public Relations Department.

Teo, You Yenn. 2019. *This Is What Inequality Looks Like: Essays by Teo You Yenn*. Singapore: Ethos Books.

Teoh, Cheng Hai. 2012. "Malaysian Corporations as Strategic Players in Southeast Asia's Palm Oil Industry." In *Palm Oil Controversy in Southeast Asia: A Transnational Perspective*. Edited by Oliver Pye, Jayati Bhattacharya, and Anthony Reid. Singapore: Institute of Southeast Asian Studies.

Thakur, Megha. 2018. "An Economic Analysis of Plight of Farmers Suicide in India." *SSRG International Journal of Economics and Management Studies* 5, no. 1 (January): 19–21.

Thomas, Hugh. 1971. *Cuba: The Pursuit of Freedom*. New York: Harper & Row.

Thomas, John. 2016. *Evangelising the Nation: Religion and the Formation of Naga Political Identity*. New Delhi: Routledge.

Thomas, Madathilparampil Mammen. 1971. "Salvation and Humanization: A Crucial Issue in the Theology of Mission for India." *International Review of Mission* 60, no. 237 (January): 25–38.

Thomas, S. 2014. "The Wonder That Is Cassava." *Guyana Chronicle*, September 29, 2014. https://guyanachronicle.com/2014/09/29/the-wonder-that-is-cassava/.

Thompson, Akola.2021. "Curried Chicken or Chicken Curry? The Debate Continues," *Loop Caribbean News* (October 15, 2021).

Thumra, Jonathan H. 2003. "The Naga Primal (Traditional) Religion and Christianity: A Theological Reflection." In *In Search of Praxis Theology for the Nagas*. Edited by V. K. Nuh. Delhi: Regency.

Tilzey, Mark. 2018. *Political Ecology, Food Regimes, and Food Sovereignty: Crisis, Resistance, and Resilience*. Coventry: Coventry University.

Tinker, Tink. 1993. *Missionary Conquest: The Gospel and Native American Cultural Genocide*. Minneapolis: Fortress Press.

________. 2008. "Christology and Colonialism: Jesus, Corn Mother, and Conquest." In *American Indian Liberation: A Theology of Sovereignty*. Maryknoll, NY: Orbis.

________. 2013. "Why I Do Not Believe in a Creator." In *Buffalo Shout, Salmon Cry: Conversations on Creation, Land Justice, and Life Together*. Edited By Steve Heinrichs. Harrisonburg, VA: Herald Press.

Tola, Miriam. 2018. "Between Pachamama and Mother Earth: Gender, Political Ontology, and the Rights of Nature in Contemporary Bolivia." *Feminist Review* 118, no. 1: 25–40.

Toussaint-Samat, Maguelonne. (1987) 2009. *A History of Food*. Translated by Anthea Bell. West Sussex, GB: Blackwell Publishers.

Tsher ing, Bkra shis, editor. 2008. *Mkha' spyod 'bras ljongs kyi gnas yig phyogs bsdebs bzhugs*. Gangtok, IND: Namgyal Institute of Tibetology and Dharamsala, Amnye Machen Institute.

United Nations World Food Program. 2018–2022. "Plurinational State of Bolivia: Annual Country Report." In *United Nations World Food Program*. Country Strategic Plan (2018–2022): 1–49.

Vaka'uta, Nāsili. 2011. *Reading Ezra 9–10 Tu'a-wise: Rethinking Biblical Interpretation in Oceania*. Atlanta: Society of Biblical Literature.

Vashum, Singtitla. 2017. "Women's Contribution in Household Economy with Special Reference to the Tangkhul Naga in Manipur." *International Journal of Research and Analytical Reviews* 4, no. 4: 45–47.

Vashum, Yangkahao. 2003. "Sources of Studying Tribal Theology." In *Tribal Theology: A Reader*. Edited by Shimreingam Shimray. Assam: TSC.

Viola, Herman J., and Carolyn Margolis. 1991. *Seeds of Change: Five Hundred Years Since Columbus*. Washington, DC: Smithsonian Institution Press.

Wallace, W. C. 2023. *The Movement of Venezuelans to the Americas and the Caribbean in the 21st Century*, 1st edition. Springer Nature Switzerland.

Walsh-Dilley, Marygold. 2019. "Religious Fragmentation, Social Disintegration? Social Networks and Evangelical Protestantism in Rural Andean Bolivia." *Qualitative Sociology* 42, no. 1: 499–520.

Warman, Arturo. 2003. *Corn & Capitalism*. Translated by Nancy L. Westrate. Chapel Hill: University of North Carolina Press.

Whitney, Robert. 2001. *State and Revolution in Cuba: Mass Mobilization and Political Change, 1920–1940*. Chapel Hill, NC: University of North Carolina Press.

Wilk, Richard, and Livia Barbosa, eds. 2012. *Rice and Beans: A Unique Dish in a Hundred Places*. Oxford: Berg Publishers.

Williams, Eric. 1942. *The Negro in the Caribbean*. Washington, DC: Associates in Negro Folk Education.

Wolf, Eric R. 2005. *A Europa e os Povos sem História*. Sao Paulo: Editora da Universidade de São Paulo.

Yannick, Fer. 2011. "Religion, Pluralism, and Conflicts in the Pacific Islands." In *The Blackwell Companion to Religion and Violence*. Edited by Andrew R. Murphy. London: Wiley & Blackwell.

Zelliot, Eleanor. 2010. "India's Dalits: Racism and Contemporary Change." *Global Dialogue* 12, no. 2 (Summer): 1–9.

Index